Baptizing Alternative Medicine

Baptizing Alternative Medicine

A Guide for the Curious But Cautious Christian

W. Michael Westbrook

Writers Club Press
New York Lincoln Shanghai

Baptizing Alternative Medicine
A Guide for the Curious But Cautious Christian

Writers Club Press
an imprint of iUniverse, Inc.

For information address:
iUniverse, Inc.
2021 Pine Lake Road, Suite 100
Lincoln, NE 68512
www.iuniverse.com

ISBN: 0-595-26568-5

Printed in the United States of America

Contents

1

WHY CHRISTIANS CAN'T IGNORE ALTERNATIVE MEDICINE

God has given us the gift of life, and it is His will that we should value that gift. Most of us do love life, so it is not surprising that if we are afflicted with a debilitating or potentially fatal illness, we will struggle mightily to restore our health. If we fail to find relief through conventional channels, we will be tempted to try almost any therapy which might make us well. This search for better health can lead us to some strange places and present us with some troubling dilemmas.

Even the neutral outsider may not know how to resolve these dilemmas. A few years ago, I was a member of a small group that met on a weekly basis for Bible study, sharing, and prayer. One evening an elegantly dressed middle aged woman joined our group. I knew her by sight from church, and had heard that she had recently been diagnosed with inoperable lung cancer.

She was quiet for most of the evening, until we began to pray. After several of the other members had contributed prayers, she suddenly spoke in a clear, steady voice. "I want to thank the Lord for the miracle of macrobiotics," she began. "I know that I have been led to this marvelous healing system, and I can tell that the cancer is already being cleansed from my body. Thank you, Lord, for showing me the way to be well again."

There was an uncomfortable silence after she finished. After a few moments, one of the other members of the group broke the tension by offering a prayer for our visitor's healing.

I found my thoughts returning to the elegant lady's situation for the rest of the evening. I knew enough about macrobiotics to be both intrigued and troubled. Macrobiotics is more than a diet. It is also a philosophical system, built on a foundation of Asian thought. Some have said that it is in fact a religion, or at least that it tries to fill the hole in the heart meant for faith. I was not at all sure that our guest's commitment was compatible with Christianity. Even if macrobiotics did not explicitly deny any of the tenets of Christian faith, the macrobiotic philosophy certainly assumed a universe that did not include, or require, a savior.

At the same time, the macrobiotic diet has been utilized by a number of individuals who have claimed remarkable remissions from "incurable" cancers. The claims are anecdotal and have not been validated by science, but they are numerous. The individual cases have not been discredited, though conventional physicians would regard them as spontaneous remissions which could not necessarily be attributed to the diet. When it is practiced correctly, the macrobiotic diet is a healthy one, low in fat and high in vegetables and unrefined grains. Even if one is skeptical about the claims of cancer "cures", a careful macrobiotic diet is probably not harmful and may even be helpful, if only by increasing the cancer patient's general nutritional status.

I was very confused about what my proper response should be. It seemed that I could make an equally sound case for quietly warning our guest that she might be involved in a dangerous cult, or for applauding her dietary discipline and her willingness to take responsibility for her own health. I resolved my dilemma by not saying anything at all. Unfortunately, our guest never returned to the group. My wife and I moved a short time later, and I never heard the end of the story. To this day, I don't know if the elegant lady fought off her cancer. I certainly hope she did.

This kind of dilemma is not unusual. Anyone who suffers from a medical condition for which the standard treatment is ineffective, expensive, or uncomfortable will eventually be faced with the question of alternative treatments. Whether the possibility is broached by a friend or relative, or we go actively searching for alternatives ourselves, sooner or later we will have to decide whether or not we are willing to go beyond conventional medicine.

However we get there, when we begin exploring the world of alternative medicine, it may seem as alien to us as a foreign country. We leave the familiar world of white coats and stethoscopes for health food stores and cramped alternative bookshops, for practitioners in jeans and treatments that sometimes don't seem medical at all.

That can be troubling. Alternative treatments can sometimes seem almost like occult practices. Sometimes, to be honest, they *are* occult practices. Anything which is clearly occult in nature should be avoided by anyone who takes the guidance of the Bible and the Church seriously. As is stated in the Catechism of the Catholic Church, "All practices of *magic* or *sorcery*, by which one attempts to tame occult powers, so as to place them at one's service and have a supernatural power over others—even if this were for the sake of restoring their health—are gravely contrary to the virtue of religion." (Catechism paragraph 2117, 513-514).

The question, of course, is where the dividing line between the acceptable and the unacceptable falls. Some who have considered the issue seriously argue that essentially all alternative medicine is so tainted that it is too spiritually dangerous to use. Among Catholic thinkers, Fr. Mitch Pacwa has cogently warned of the theological dangers of the "New Age". Among evangelical Protestants, books such as The Hidden Agenda suggest that much alternative medicine is non-Christian or even anti-Christian, and may tempt the faithful away from a reliance on Christ.

The dangers are certainly real. Nonetheless, I would respectfully disagree with these authors. Alternative medicine is a mixture of good and bad, and the good is good enough that the Church can't afford to discard it. I would propose a parallel case. During the Middle Ages, Christian Europe re-encountered many works of Aristotle which had been preserved by Muslim scholars during the centuries that they were lost in the West.

The rediscovery of Aristotle by Europe caused an immediate furor. Aristotle had always been one of the foundational authorities of Western civilization, and these "new" works were clearly works of genius. At the same time, they were just as obviously pagan. Aristotle's assumptions were not Christian assumptions. He understood the universe to be pre-existent and without beginning or end, rather than a created thing. His discussions of the goals of human life and the sources of human satisfaction weren't anti-Christian, exactly, but they certainly didn't include the God who was teaching the Jews to rely on Him during the same period that Aristotle wrote. Aristotle brought to a sharp point the conflict between "Athens" and "Jerusalem" that had always been implicit in the Western tradition.

It was the great achievement of St. Thomas Aquinas to "baptize" Aristotle in such a way that he could be accepted by the medieval church. By keeping what was true and abandoning or adapting the rest, St. Thomas produced the great synthesis which still shapes Catholic theology today. Simply being pagan didn't mean that Aristotle was always wrong, but it took a brilliant theologian like St. Thomas to see that. In the same way, if there is anything of value in alternative medicine, it can and should be adapted for use by Christians who wish to aid the suffering or who are suffering themselves.

Is there anything of value in the confusing array of therapies, theories, and techniques collectively known as alternative medicine? Does alternative medicine work?

It is impossible to give a single, simple answer to that question. Each therapy must be judged on its own merits. If it can be demonstrated that chiropractic is an effective treatment for lower back pain, this says nothing about the efficacy of shark cartilage for cancer. It is important to keep this in mind, because alternative medicine is one of those controversial issues that tends to produce very polarized positions. Either alternative medicine is pure superstition and a rejection of science, or alternative medicine could heal the world's worst scourges if it wasn't for the monopolistic conspiracies of the A.M.A. and its minions. Both of these extremes are false.

Instead, it is safe to say that some alternative medicine works, and some does not. Some alternative medicine works very well, better than more orthodox treatments for the same condition. Some alternative medicine doesn't work at all and may even be actively dangerous, though this is far less common than one might believe listening to apologists for regular medicine. Later chapters will consider some specific alternatives in detail, but one general point can be made. People on both sides of the alternative divide frequently assume that the distinction between conventional and alternative medicine is a distinction between scientific medicine and medicine which does not bear this imprimatur. Once one has accepted (incorrectly) that conventional medicine is the only scientific medicine, it is an easy step to the belief that conventional medicine is the only medicine with proven effectiveness.

To be "scientific" in the culture of medicine means, among other things, that a given therapy has a clearly understood mechanism of action. A therapy which has been repeatedly demonstrated to be effective can still be considered unscientific and therefore unacceptable if the consensus of the scientific community holds that it is irrational or impossible. The best example of this is homeopathy, a system which has been producing successful cures for nearly two hundred years. Homeopathy treats patients with tiny doses of substances which, if given to a healthy person, would produce the same symptoms as those that the patient is experiencing because of illness. The basic principle is "like cures like".

The most problematic element of this system for modern science is the preparation of the medicines. Homeopathic remedies are produced by a process of repeated dilution that proceeds so far that there are probably no molecules of the original medicine left in the resulting solution. Homeopaths believe that by "potentizing" the solution at each stage, the remedy retains the medicinal power of the original substance without the potential for harm. Potentization involves vigorous shaking or pounding of the water and alcohol medium.

Conventional science knows of no mechanism by which homeopathic remedies could maintain any activity in the body after their dilution. For nearly two hundred years, the remedies have been mocked as pure placebos, harmless but utterly useless in the face of serious disease. For anyone who believes in the power of reason to understand the natural world, it is tempting to dismiss homeopathy as one of the sillier aberrations the human mind has produced. There is only one problem with this simple, comfortable solution. Homeopathy works.

This conclusion is so unbelievable to reasonable people that it has been repeatedly tested with the tools of orthodox science. Though not all of the trials have produced clear, unambiguous results, taken as a whole the outcome of these experiments has been positive enough that the authors of a review article in the British Medical Journal stated "Based on this evidence, we would be ready to accept that homeopathy can be efficacious, if only the mechanism of action were more plausible" (Kleijnen et al. 321). The scientific community rejects homeopathy, not because it doesn't work, but because it doesn't make sense. This is not a negligible issue, but it is certainly a *different* issue from what most people believe to be the core of the orthodox critique. Frequently this difference is fudged, as if "we don't understand this" meant the same thing as "this isn't happening".

Though homeopathy provides the clearest example, other forms of alternative medicine are in the same position. Chiropractic has demonstrated its effectiveness for musculoskeletal complaints (Assendelft et al. 1942-1948), but it has been vilified for decades because its foundational theory seems irrational to mainstream physicians and scientists.

Traditional Chinese medicine has begun to edge its way into scientific respectability, but only with the Chinese understanding of its action stripped away and a new explanation substituted. The new scientific explanation explains less and has less predictive power than the Chinese version, but it fits better with the rest of Western science. This is not to say that the Western explanation is wrong, but that it has certainly been selected on the basis of criteria more complicated than "Is this true?" or "Does this work?"

If we are willing to examine alternative medicine with only the single question "Does this work?" in mind, we will find a number of therapies about which we can answer affirmatively, even if it is not clear how or why they work. Perhaps any beneficial effect is a pure placebo response, produced by the individual's belief in the power of the medicine rather than by any intrinsic activity of the medicine itself. As Andrew Weil has pointed out, a beneficial effect is a beneficial effect (Weil 218). If healing has taken place, let's be grateful and rejoice. Assuming that the therapy we used violates no moral law, then we can worry about the mechanism of action when we are relaxed, happy, and well.

If in fact there are alternative therapies with the power to heal, then these therapies have a role to play in relieving suffering. It should go without saying that Christians have an interest in relieving suffering—an interest that should be far more compelling than any need to remain respectable or "scientific". Our Lord was hardly respectable during His earthly ministry, and His healings were certainly not scientific if science requires that we understand every detail of God's "mechanism of action".

Instead, we follow a Lord who was frequently mysterious but always compassionate. Our own compassion should encourage us to explore any healing tool or technique which is both lawful and effective. If a therapy heals the sick and does not violate any ordinance of the Church or Scripture, then it may have a role to play regardless of whether or not we understand exactly how it works.

Indeed, in some ways the kinds of therapies which we find among alternative medicine provide a better fit with Christianity than does conventional medicine. One of the most consistent characteristics of alternative approaches is an emphasis on the whole person. This emphasis is so consistent that it is sometimes taken to be the defining characteristic of non-mainstream approaches, as in the use of the term "holistic medicine" to serve as a synonym for alternative or complementary medicine. Though there are exceptions, this generalization is not far wrong. Where conventional medicine focuses on finding the "part that broke", alternative medicine concerns itself with the person who is ill.

This is one of the chief sources of friction between the alternative community and regular M.D.s. Since alternative practitioners are interested in strengthening the whole person to resist illness, they frequently use therapies that affect functions or systems with no direct relationship to the illness itself, if these appear to be areas of weakness impeding the body's coordinated response. For instance, chiropractors believe that they can remove impediments to the free transmission of messages through the nervous system and thereby release the body's innate power to heal. This appears irrational to the conventional M.D., who asks why asthma or irritable bowel syndrome should respond to spinal manipulation. It is revealing that there are a growing number of M.D.s who are willing to consider a role for chiropractic, *if* chiropractors will limit themselves to the treatment of musculoskeletal problems of the back and neck. In other words, "real" medicine is something like being a car mechanic, where the goal is to find the malfunctioning part and fix it. A broken axle doesn't respond to a new paint job or a tuneup, and a migraine headache won't respond to an adjustment of the spine.

It should be clear that human beings are not cars. Our parts are tied together through so many subtle channels of communication and mutually interacting feedback loops that it should not be surprising if a stimulus applied to one part of the body has a multitude of effects in other parts of the body. This web of interactions includes the mind, that glorious seat of awareness and will which has no counterpart in the purely mechanical world which so many M.D.s appear to inhabit.

Human beings are most accurately regarded as persons, rather than mechanisms. A person is a single, integrated whole, alive and aware and capable both of influencing and being influenced by the world around them. Rather than being fixed, a person heals. Healing is an active process which requires that the body regulate and coordinate its functions. Being fixed, or, to use the preferred phrase in medicine, being cured, is a passive process requiring only that the sick individual submit to the ministrations of the proper expert.

Christianity addresses persons, not mechanisms. Our Lord did not die on the cross to serve wind-up toys. When He calls us to repent and return to Him, it is clear that He has given us the awareness and freedom to be morally responsible agents. He has given us the gift of personhood.

Unfortunately, all too often we surrender the dignity of personhood as soon as it comes time to tend to our physical health. We maintain a strange pair of conflicting perspectives—we are persons before God but a set of parts before our physician. In my experience, alternative practitioners are much better at treating people as persons than are conventional M.D.s.

This includes an aspect of personhood which has been all but written out of regular medicine—the realm of the spirit. In keeping with the unstated rules of the culture of science, medicine regards spiritual concerns as irrelevant to the body's physiological functioning. The body is to be understood with the tools of science, and by definition science limits itself to the purely natural. This is not to say that scientists can't be religious. Many scientists are people of deep personal faith. Nonetheless, when in their professional capacity they are asked to provide a scientific explanation of an event, they cannot respond "God did it" unless they wish to step outside the range of explanations which are acceptable to the scientific community.

To give the scientific community its just due, this lack of attention to the spiritual is generally not intended to imply that the spiritual doesn't exist. It is instead an attempt to limit science to those questions which the tools of science can legitimately answer, while leaving theology to the theologians. Unfortunately, the world does not divide neatly along disciplinary boundaries, and this is particularly true in medicine. If we attempt to exclude any role for the spirit in our understanding of the body, we end up with a false picture of what human beings are and how human beings function.

We also end up with a false picture of God. Dietrich Bonhoeffer warned of the modern tendency to imagine a "God of the gaps" (Bonhoeffer 190-191). This is a God whose only role is to provide an explanation for whatever phenomena have not yet been explained by science. The problem with a God of the gaps is that as science closes the gaps, God disappears.

The relationship of the biblical God to His creation is both more intimate and more subtle than that of the modernist God. There are no purely natural events for which God has no interest or concern. "Are not two sparrows sold for a penny? Yet not one of them will fall to the ground apart from your father," (Matthew 10:29). Christian thinkers have generally used the term "providence" to describe God's ongoing care of creation.

Providence does not conflict with the working of nature as described by science. Providence is, in fact, the source and substrate of nature. God wants His care of the natural world to unfold with a regularity which can be discerned by human reason. We call the regularities we see "the laws of nature", but they are more properly thought of as the laws by which nature is ruled. Nature is the object of the laws, not the lawmaker. There is only One who holds that position.

We tend to think of the physical universe as reality, and spiritual concerns as somehow apart from or even incidental to that reality. We conceive of our bodies and our spirits as following parallel but nonintersecting paths. Though this is often believed to be the Christian understanding of human nature, in fact it is a product of the rationalism which we have inherited from the Enlightenment. The ancient Hebrews viewed human beings as indivisibly one, matter and spirit intertwined so thoroughly that they cannot be teased apart.

This means that chains of cause and effect can run across the divide between matter and spirit. Spiritual causes, like prayer, can have material effects, like the healing of physical illness. The chain can also run in the other direction. Events that appear to be purely material can have spiritual consequences.

This last assertion may be shocking to some, so accustomed have we become to locking our spiritual lives away in a compartment separate from the rest of our existence. Catholic Christians steeped in the sacramental theology of the Church are quite comfortable with the idea that matter, like bread and wine, can serve as a vehicle for spirit. Protestants, on the other hand, may find this idea troubling, even idolatrous or occult in nature.

It may be helpful to remember that all of the sundered branches of Christendom, without exception, teach that there is at least one channel through which matter can affect spirit. That channel is sin. Food approached gluttonously or sex approached lustfully leave real stains on the soul.

These examples show how impossible it is to separate matter and spirit in the real world we live in. Both the material object of sin, like a cheesecake, and the spiritual predisposition to consume it gluttonously participate in producing the resulting sin. In the same way we need to remember that all healing is in some sense spiritual healing. There is no part of us that is untouched by spirit. There is no purely material body that we can drop off at the doctor's office to have fixed while our souls continue on their way untouched. All illness, and all healing, have a meaning for us, and meaning is a spiritual quality.

The willingness of alternative practitioners to attend to this meaning is one of the primary reasons for their continued success in the face of the organized hostility of the medical establishment. Sufferers need to have an explanation and a context for their illness that will enable them to integrate that illness with the rest of their lives. In some cases, this need can be so compelling that patients will continue to patronize a practitioner who can provide such a context even if he or she can't cure, or even affect, the illness itself. In traditional pre-industrial cultures where the power to affect the course of illness is limited, this is the primary role of the healer. Modern men and women have not lost the need for meaning just because scientific medicine has concluded that meaning no longer falls within its sphere of responsibility.

Unfortunately, meanings are not interchangeable. It makes a difference whether we view our sufferings as a redemptive sharing in the cross of Christ or as a mindless turn of the wheel of karma. The ill need help to find a way of understanding and transcending their condition, and this makes them vulnerable to those who would present themselves as saviors, medical or otherwise. Alternative practitioners are not priests or pastors, but they often function as such. We cannot abandon the suffering to their ministrations without guidance.

This then is the final reason why Christendom cannot ignore alternative medicine. We have brothers and sisters, both Christian and non-Christian, who are suffering. Many of the suffering have illnesses for which there are no reliable answers in conventional medicine. These people *are* turning to alternative medicine.

This is frequently a reasonable decision. There are effective therapies among the alternatives. Alternative practitioners in general work with a more sophisticated model of human nature than do conventional physicians. They are also more comfortable with life's spiritual dimension. Given these strengths, it seems obvious that for some people in some circumstances, alternative medicine may be the best available option.

Unfortunately, it is an option that brings with it a unique set of dangers. It is one of the strengths of conventional medicine that it is regularized and standardized. Whether or not conventional treatment is the best available approach to your condition, at least you know what you are going to get. This isn't true for alternative medicine. When you seek out an alternative practitioner, you may get superb cutting edge therapy or you may get dangerous occult mumbo jumbo. It may be difficult to tell the difference between the two.

The good in alternative medicine is good enough that any recommendation to simply avoid it is irresponsible, the rough equivalent of prohibiting dancing or alcohol because they can be abused. The Church must recognize that its interests are not identical with those of any particular approach to medicine. If alternative medicine sometimes teaches bad theology, the mechanistic model of conventional medicine has a built-in bias against any theology whatsoever. The Church must stand apart from any single medical sect in order to provide moral and spiritual guidance for all. If individual Christians seek healing outside standard medicine, they must not be driven beyond the pale for this. Instead, the Church must be there to provide a framework for discernment. In the sometimes wild and wooly world of alternative medicine, we may need all the discernment we can get.

2

WHY CHRISTIANS CAN'T ACCEPT ALTERNATIVE MEDICINE AS THEY FIND IT

Stepping into the world of alternative medicine is like stepping into a howling wilderness. There are riches hidden here and there, but to find them one must first avoid the wolves and the bears that wait for the unwary. The dangers are both physical and spiritual. The most likely difficulty one may encounter is simply receiving an ineffective treatment.

It is an unfortunate fact that many alternatives just don't work, or don't work very well. This is not to imply that the practitioners who employ them are deliberate quacks or con artists. In my experience, the overwhelming majority of people who work with alternative therapies are deeply sincere. Indeed, their commitment to what might be termed the alternative worldview is so profound that it amounts to a religious commitment. This is a subject that will be addressed later in this chapter. Nonetheless, despite their sincerity, many of them work with techniques that have little power to heal.

This is true for a variety of reasons. One is an unfortunate side effect of a holistic perspective. Almost by definition, holism and careful analytical thinking are often at odds. Analytical thinking involves uncovering component parts of a problem, taking them apart and solving them step by step with careful attention to the linear relationships of cause

14

and effect. Holism avoids this kind of reductionist analysis to focus on things as they are, with all of their complexities and ambiguities. While this does in some ways present a more complete picture of reality, it also excludes some of the most powerful tools of critical thinking. Insofar as members of the alternative community are committed to a purely holistic perspective, they may be unable to perform the kinds of analysis that would cause them to discard some techniques as ineffective.

There is also an anarchic quality to the alternative community. This unwillingness to accept or exercise authority is frequently a part of a deeply felt set of philosophical commitments, though it is probably inevitable just by virtue of having stepped beyond the reach of the control mechanisms of bureaucratic regular medicine. Though these control mechanisms are frequently employed too vigorously, they do at least ensure that conventional medicine is capable of expelling incompetents and, however slowly and fitfully, moving beyond demonstrably false ideas. In the alternative community, no person or practice is ever rejected.

Indeed, it is one of the ironies of the present medical scene that obsolete conventional techniques are now available as alternatives. Before the advent of the microbiological era, conventional medicine was driven by a mechanical metaphor that reduced the body to a set of pumps and tubes. Illness was the result of a loss of tone in the body's many muscular pipes. This could be restored by a variety of means, including the use of enemas and purgatives to stimulate the colon.

We are all grateful that conventional medicine has lost its fascination with bowel function. As regular medicine moved beyond this idea, however, the alternative community took it up with enthusiasm and even extended it. It is now an article of faith in some alternative circles that most people's colons are caked with masses of putrefying feces that are not expelled by ordinary bowel movements. It is asserted that these deposits can only be removed through bowel cleansing regimens involving herbal laxatives and enemas. Sometimes the regimens include high colonics, a form of enema administered by machine which forces water into the colon under pressure. I have seen books for sale in health food stores with glossy color photographs of six to ten foot long rubbery looking masses supposedly removed from sick people by these techniques.

The problem with these assertions is that regular medicine moved beyond purgatives and cathartics for a reason. The model of human physiological function upon which these therapies were based was oversimplified and insufficient to explain most illness. Subsequent science has repeatedly confirmed this. It is worth remembering that M.D.s look into colons all the time, without seeing the fecal deposits claimed by colonic therapists. Constipation simply is not the cause of most human disease.

Why then has this form of therapy survived in alternative circles long after it was discarded by conventional medicine? One simple answer has already been alluded to. There is no mechanism in place to remove this or any other ineffective therapy from the alternative armamentarium. In addition, since the toxic buildup in the colon is usually attributed to processed foods, lack of exercise, and chemical exposure, the theory of fecal overload fits with a consistent sense in the alternative community that the modern world is a Bad Thing. Finally, the techniques survive because they do occasionally cure illness.

This last may seem a surprising assertion, but there are many testimonials to this effect. Indeed, one of the major difficulties in sorting effective therapies from ineffective ones is that it is possible to find testimonials for almost anything. This is one reason why conventional physicians tend to dismiss the successes of alternative medicine as examples of the placebo effect.

Sometimes this is true, though it would be false to assume that this means that the therapies have no activity whatsoever. Andrew Weil has proposed that many remedies, both conventional and otherwise, function as "active placebos" (Weil 219-233). An active placebo is a treatment which has a real, potentially therapeutic effect on the body but which produces its primary benefit by stimulating the body's innate healing power through the placebo effect. Though Weil tends to conceive of this healing power as primarily mediated by the mind, it is also possible that the dynamic complexity of the mind/body system may allow a purely physical stimulus to initiate a healing response even if it doesn't really address the cause of the illness. Sometimes any change of state is enough to break a logjam.

This kind of response, though, isn't consistent enough to be relied upon, especially in the face of serious illness. There are a huge number of alternative therapies that produce measurable physiological changes in healthy directions, but which simply aren't very potent when compared to drugs or surgery. All of the various forms of massage therapy are superb at producing profound relaxation. This makes them very useful adjunct therapies for stress related conditions, but I would not rely on massage alone to treat heart disease, for example.

This is true even for esoteric variations of massage which claim the ability to treat serious disease through channels ignored by Western science. Foot reflexology, for instance, postulates that zones on the feet correspond to the various organ systems of the body, so that a specialized form of foot massage can affect the function of the internal organs and produce healing. Reflexologists can point to the usual catalog of testimonials and even a few published studies in support of their therapy. Unfortunately, none of the studies give clear evidence for the objective reality of the reflexology zones. The most parsimonious explanation for reflexology's successes is that foot massage is very relaxing, and sometimes relaxation is enough.

There are innumerable examples of alternative therapies whose primary effect is to make people feel good. Aromatherapy, which relies on fragrant essential oils, can produce marvelously sensual experiences, but there is no strong evidence that it has any intrinsic healing power more potent than a warm bath, a good meal, or a vacation. There is nothing wrong with making people feel good, and these therapies have real applications for this reason alone. Massage and aromatherapy have been used in hospital intensive care units to reduce the intense stress which a stay in an I.C.U. can produce. Nonetheless, it would hardly be prudent to turn off the monitors and take down the I.V. in the hope that a little lavender oil rubbed into the temples will serve as well.

If the therapeutic anarchy in the alternative community simply meant that people might have to sort through a variety of possibilities to find the truly effective therapies, then this would probably be a tolerable level of hazard. Though therapies with little or no activity are common, truly dangerous therapies are rare. Of the therapies already discussed in this chapter, only bowel cleansing regimens are likely to do real harm. These regimens, especially when practiced for long periods, can destroy the normal rhythm of the bowel and produce severe laxative dependence. High colonic machines can transmit intestinal parasites from patient to patient and can damage the muscular wall of the colon.

Massage, reflexology, and aromatherapy, on the other hand, are clearly safe when competently performed. If nothing else, they reduce stress and are pleasant to receive. This alone may produce benefits in a variety of conditions. The only problem is that one of these therapies, reflexology, teaches as fact certain things about the human body which are almost certainly untrue. Is there any reason to be concerned about a therapy like this, a therapy which is both comforting and wrong?

Here we enter the realm of spiritual dangers. The therapies in themselves are usually not dangerous, but the attitudes they engender can be. The therapeutic anarchy of the alternative community is frequently defended by an appeal to a wholesale epistemological anarchy, relativism run riot. Holistic healers prefer to speak of realities and truths rather than reality and truth. Many in the alternative community have been influenced by the common New Age belief that reality is a construction of the observer and that there are as many realities as there are people to perceive them.

This is certainly a convenient doctrine when one is promoting a therapy which cannot bear close analysis, but it has a number of problems. Not the least of these is that the doctrine is simply false. It stems from a misunderstanding of modern physics coupled with a bastard-ized form of Hinduism and Buddhism. The tenet of physics which is frequently invoked in defense of relativism is the Heisenberg Uncertainty Principle.

Werner Heisenberg demonstrated in 1927 that it was impossible to measure both the position and momentum of a particle at the same time and derive exact values for both measurements. The act of measuring one value affects the other. The observer cannot eliminate the effect of the act of observation.

This is a remarkable truth. It means that we can no longer accept the clockwork universe imagined by the thinkers of the Enlightenment, in which all events could in theory be predicted if we knew the position and velocity of every particle that existed. Since this kind of knowledge is prohibited by the very structure of the universe, a degree of indeterminacy seems built in to reality. While this is comforting to those of us who prefer not to be perfectly predictable automatons, it is important to note that it is an indeterminacy with limits.

The observer measuring the position of a particle affects its momentum, but the particle still has a reality independent of the observer. The observer cannot choose to see five particles, or no particles at all. If quantum physics has proved that any description of reality is essentially arbitrary, then no one has gotten the word to the physicists. They are still hard at work attempting to construct a single comprehensive description of a unitary reality.

The second doctrine used in defense of New Age relativism is the Eastern concept of maya, or illusion. Both Hindus and Buddhists believe that the material world, the world of forms in which we live our daily lives, is essentially illusory. Though the two traditions understand this somewhat differently and work out the consequences in different ways, both traditions agree that everyday reality is only contingently real and that it is a distraction from the Absolute, Reality with a capital R. Both traditions also see a role for consciousness in sustaining the world of forms.

Whatever we think of this idea in its original form (and it is clearly not a Christian idea), it has just as clearly been distorted when it is put into the service of the infinitely malleable consciousness-driven universe of New Age thinkers. Maya is not the final level of reality in Eastern thought, but it is not subject to unlimited editing at the whim of the observer either. Some things are true of it and others are not.

When the alternative community attempts to avoid the issue of effectiveness by insisting on a multiplicity of realities, or when they invoke the power of consciousness as if it were a deity, they are offering us a simple-minded epistemology. It is an epistemology that tends to short-circuit any serious examination of the meaning of human life by insisting at the outset that no single answer is possible, let alone sufficient.

There is one all-sufficient answer to the problem of meaning, and He is Christ. This is not a work of Christian apologetics, so it is not our purpose to demonstrate the sufficiency of Christianity. It is our purpose to warn those who already know the Living Lord that they must guard against those who would undercut our reliance on the Savior with Pilate's question: "What is truth?"

This is not the only hostile question which will be posed to Christians who enter the world of alternative medicine. Alternative medicine frequently comes embedded in a distinctly non-Christian and sometimes overtly anti-Christian culture. Health food stores never sell Bibles or catechisms, but they frequently stock New Age titles or works of Eastern spirituality that are only peripherally about health. Alternative magazines run articles extolling Buddhism or Native American religion as an answer to the empty materialism of the West.

Alternative thinkers almost never acknowledge that there is an authentic Western spiritual tradition that is very much alive today. If they do mention Christianity, it is in disparaging, dismissive tones. I have heard it casually asserted that most gynecological difficulties occur in women who were raised Catholic, and who were therefore sexually abused by the Church's teaching. A major national health magazine ran a glowing profile of Matthew Fox, the renegade Dominican priest who has been silenced by the Vatican because he insists on teaching a "creation spirituality" which denies many of the bedrock doctrines of Christianity (Knaster 21-24). Historic supernatural Christianity, the faith of the fathers, is almost never treated as a serious option in alternative literature.

One problem for these writers is Christianity's exclusivity. In Jesus' own words, "No one comes to the Father but by me," (John 14.6). This exclusive claim is central to Christianity, and it is understood in the alternative community as a repudiation of the warm fuzzy inclusiveness which they prize so deeply. The only truth which the alternative community cannot accept is a truth which claims to be The Truth.

A whole series of unconvincing criticisms are spun off from this reflexive resistance to binding truth claims. It is argued that Christian exclusivity is the reason for the oppression of native peoples, for the rape of the environment, and even for the generally poor taste of middle America. If we would just give up our silly claim to know the Way, the Truth, and the Life, then Christian priests could join the gurus and shamans in the New Age spiritual supermarket and everyone would be nonjudgmentally content.

Unfortunately, this is the one claim we cannot surrender. Jesus didn't die on the cross just for those who find the gesture personally meaningful, but for all human beings. We don't have to condemn all non-Christians to hell. We just need to affirm that if human beings are saved, they are saved by Christ, whether they know it or not. Without this central assertion, we have taken Christ out of Christianity and we are no longer dealing with the same religion.

This is the hidden danger of alternative inclusiveness. What appears at the outset to be simple politeness can rapidly become a religious alternative in itself—a new faith which maintains the forms of Christianity for those who find them appealing but which has lost any reliance on the Savior. It is the central claim of Christianity that human beings cannot reach God unaided, and that Christ is the way God has provided for us to reach Him. If human beings can reach God by the various spiritual disciplines espoused in the alternative community, then the Christian claim is false.

If this is our choice, then as Christians we are obligated to turn our backs on the alternative option. We cannot allow anything to stand between us and complete reliance on the Lord. If alternative medicine cannot be separated from New Age paganism, if the various available therapies grow out of and depend upon anti-Christian assumptions, then alternative medicine must be rejected.

Luckily, these are not our only two options. Though it is true that alternative medicine and New Age religious thinking frequently travel together, they can be readily distinguished. In many cases the connection amounts to little more than a historical accident, a remnant of the counterculture's uncritical enthusiasm for all things anti-establishment during the 1960s. Most of the major alternative traditions have long histories that predate their connection with the New Age by decades or even centuries.

For instance, during the Nineteenth Century homeopathy was practiced by highly educated conventional physicians. Though it was always the method of a minority, in its early decades its growth was so rapid and its success so apparent that it seemed for a few years that it might well become "regular medicine". This didn't happen for a variety of reasons. Homeopaths couldn't offer any explanation for the success of their therapy. For all its power, homeopathy was difficult to do and results were frequently unpredictable. Worst of all, homeopathy started to seem old fashioned, as rapidly growing scientific knowledge seemed to offer the possibility of more direct intervention into disease processes.

During homeopathy's long decline, it was kept alive by deeply conservative physicians whose adherence to homeopathy was a sign of their deference to authority, not their resistance to it. Several observers have noted that this conservatism extended to political and religious matters as well as medical (Grossinger 118-119). These distinguished physicians would have been shocked if anyone had suggested to them that there would someday be a link between homeopathy and the anarchic paganism of the New Age movement.

Similarly, the founder of osteopathy, Andrew Taylor Still, began as a conventional physician. When he abandoned drug therapy for manipulation of the body's bones, muscles, and other structures, he was indeed regarded as a heretic by other physicians, but there was never a hint that this was anything other than a dispute over medical technique. Still was as reductionist and mechanical in his approach as any other physician—indeed, he began to emphasize manipulation precisely because of his view of the body as a machine.

When Still's followers abandoned their resistance to drugs, they also lost their alternative taint. As long as they used standard therapies, osteopaths were regarded as mainstream. Over the last few decades, some young osteopaths have re-emphasized manipulation. This alone has been sufficient to place them right back in the alternative community. No New Age religious commitment was required.

It is true that the connection between alternative medicine and New Age paganism is not wholly arbitrary, but it is important to understand the nature of the connection. It is definitely not true that one is a surrogate for the other, or that alternative medicine is a sort of Trojan Horse designed to infiltrate the New Age into the minds of the unsuspecting. Instead, the two movements tend to travel together because certain ideas and assumptions are common to both.

Both movements prize the authority of an individual's experience over any kind of institutional authority. Both share an interest in the development of the individual, whether this is conceived of in spiritual or purely physical ways. Both maintain a somewhat jaundiced view of mainstream Western culture, particularly its technological focus. Both are willing to accept the truth of a variety of phenomena with no currently acceptable scientific explanation. And, as previously discussed, both prefer holism to any kind of reductionist analysis. Holism includes a desire and a willingness to find spiritual meaning in experience, especially experience that isn't traditionally religious.

Obviously, not all of these ideas can be uncritically accepted. Christians are a people under authority, and a reflexive resistance to authority is frequently nothing more than a temptation to sin. Self development as an end in itself is simply not the proper goal of human life. Spiritual holism can become a pantheism that denies God's transcendence. Perhaps most troubling of all, the interest in the paranormal can easily become occultism.

At the same time, these are abuses of the ideas in question. Any idea can be abused, and it is unfair to judge an idea by its abuses. If we do, then we see only a caricature of the original thought. Alternative thinking is not anti-Christian by its nature (though both Christians and alternative thinkers may find this surprising). For instance, it is possible to distinguish legitimate authority instituted by God and purely human authority, so not all resistance to authority is automatically wrong. One can easily imagine an unjust, abusive authority that one would be morally obligated to resist. Recent history has given us more than one example of this kind of authority. We cannot condemn alternative thinkers simply because they lack respect for authority, since under certain circumstances this has been characteristic of the saints as well.

Similarly, if an interest in spiritual development does not involve an explicit denial of Christian doctrine and if it has an end beyond the self, then it is hard to condemn it out of hand. We are all called to spiritual growth. It should be obvious that an interest in spiritual growth is as appropriate for a Christian as it is for any New Age seeker.

We are left with the problem of occultism. This is where the most serious difficulties with alternative medicine arise, for it is unquestionably true that some alternative therapies are occult in nature. Chapter Four will consider some ways to distinguish these occult practices. There are some observers of the alternative scene who argue that *all* alternatives are based on a magical rather than a scientific world view and that they therefore qualify as occultism. Is this a legitimate concern?

It is worth remembering that science is not a finished product. There is not yet a scientific explanation for every event in the natural world. In the nineteenth century, reports by lay people that they had seen rocks falling from the sky were dismissed by the scientific community. These reports seemed so ridiculous that it was assumed that they were the product of ignorance, superstition, or hallucination. Today, of course, we recognize meteorites as a purely natural phenomenon. It does not belittle the achievements of science to admit that there may be other as yet unexplained forces or objects that science has not yet addressed.

Many alternative therapies appear, in Richard Grossinger's phrase, to be "the medicine of an unknown science," (Grossinger 2). In some cases, this means that proponents of a given therapy have suggested a plausible natural mechanism for their therapy which has not yet been tested or confirmed by mainstream science. Linus Pauling argued that human beings suffered from a deleterious genetic mutation that prevented us, in contrast to almost all of the rest of the animal kingdom, from synthesizing our own vitamin C. He was convinced that this justified supplementing vitamin C in the quantities appropriate to a physiological metabolite rather than a vitamin. Pauling may have been right or he may have been wrong, but in either case it seems unreasonable to accuse him of occultism.

Other cases are more ambiguous. Not all alternatives have a plausible mechanism of action. This does not necessarily mean that these alternatives are therefore clearly occult. Occultism involves the attempt to manipulate supernatural forces with the human will. If we extend this definition to include anything we don't understand, then we lose sight of the real, identifiable sin that underlies occultism—the human attempt to usurp the prerogatives of God. Not everything that is inexplicable is sinful.

As an example, homeopathic pharmacy involves repeated dilution and shaking of the remedy. This process is no different in character from other forms of chemical manipulation in pharmacy, except that it produces inexplicable results. It is not a ritual, and it is not an attempt to invoke magical or supernatural powers. If homeopathy works (and there are many controlled trials to indicate that it does), then some natural process is responsible for its success.

Individual homeopaths have sometimes written that the preparation of the remedies somehow releases the "spirit" or the "energy" of the original substance. This is an attempt to produce an explanation after the fact. In the same way, those of us who aren't physicists might say that an atomic bomb releases the energy of the atom, without having any real idea of how that happens. Our explanation reveals that we do not yet have a deep understanding of the process, but it does not imply that the process is occult.

In fact, in the case of homeopathic pharmacy, the process was discovered empirically in the best tradition of experimental science. Samuel Hahnemann, the founder of homeopathy, discovered the technique of potentization while experimenting with ways to reduce the initial aggravation of symptoms sometimes caused by the similar remedy in larger doses. He stuck with the technique because it worked, but we know from his writings that even he was troubled by the degree of dilution he was producing in the higher potencies (Grossinger 92). Just as with Pauling, Hahnemann may have been wrong, but it seems unfair to call him a magician simply because he produced anomalous results.

There are some elements of the typical holistic or alternative perspective that are also present in a magical world view. The religious believer needs to be careful about pointing fingers, however, because these are also a feature of traditional Christianity. Alternative healers generally believe that the universe has meaning and purpose, and that life is qualitatively different from non-life. Living beings possess something, whether it be a life force, a spirit, or a soul, that makes them more than simple matter. It is this life force that enables them to grow, adapt, change, and heal.

This belief is contemptuously dismissed by modern scientists as "vitalism". It is believed to have been discredited in the nineteenth century with the discovery that the chemicals in the body are the same as the constituents of the nonliving world. Many in the evangelical community are convinced that vitalism is a variety of occultism. Vitalism has a far more respectable pedigree than this, however, since it was the nearly universal belief of all mankind, including Christendom, until the rise of purely materialist science beginning in the Enlightenment. It is the belief that living things are nothing but meat machines which would have struck the early Church fathers as shocking, not vitalism. Though we must not attempt to manipulate the soul or spirit through magical means, there is nothing wrong with believing that it exists, or that it plays a role in healing.

It seems, then, that we can neither completely dismiss nor uncritically accept the foundational ideas of most alternative medicine. Alternative medicine is a mixture of effective, somewhat effective, and ineffective therapies which usually present themselves through the medium of a culture whose assumptions can be troubling. That culture has connections to the counter-culture of the 60s and the New Age movement of the present though it is not identical with either of these. It is generally hostile to authority, universal truth claims and sometimes to Christianity itself, though it is perhaps more accurate to call it non-Christian rather than anti-Christian. This is usually a matter of tone, since the explicit denial of Christian doctrine is rare.

As an example of how this difference in tone works itself out in practice, we might consider the perfectionism implicit in much alternative medicine. It is not uncommon in alternative writing to imply that if we all ate natural foods, took vitamin supplements, exercised and meditated every day, no one would ever get sick. I have even seen it said that if world leaders would submit to the ministrations of a massage therapist every day, international conflicts would be more swiftly resolved and a new age of peace would dawn. In general, alternative thinkers underestimate the tenacity of evil and overestimate the human ability to control or eliminate it by their own efforts. This perspective is not anti-Christian, but it certainly has very little in common with the Christian understanding of sin and evil.

It simply is not true that all or even most human illness is the result of a failure to adopt a healthy lifestyle. Sickness and death are a product of the fallen state of both the world we live in and our own natures. The suffering and pain human beings inevitably experience will never be eliminated by any combination of medical techniques, whether conventional or alternative. Only a savior can bring salvation.

Frequently, alternative thinkers who attempt to explain disease sound very much like Jesus' disciples in John 9:1-2. "As he walked along, he saw a man blind from birth. His disciples asked him, 'Rabbi, who sinned, this man or his parents, that he was born blind?' Jesus answered, 'Neither this man nor his parents sinned; he was born blind so that God's works might be revealed in him.'" The understanding of sin has certainly changed, but it remains true that many in the alternative community have a tendency to point fingers. If someone is sick, someone is at fault. If it isn't the individual, then it is the individual's parents. If it isn't the parents, then it must be the corporations who poison our water and feed us processed foods. *Someone* must be to blame.

The Church must remind the alternative community and the larger culture of Jesus' response to the accusation implied by the disciples' question. Sickness and death are not personal failures. They are a part of the human condition. And they are intended to lead us to God.

The alternative community needs the balancing influence of the Gospel, to remind its members that the quest for health and healing must not become an end in itself. Without the Gospel, alternative medicine will inevitably become an idol. With the Gospel, alternative medicine can be gleaned for those valuable techniques that do have the power to alleviate suffering.

3

THE THEOLOGY OF HEALING

It is unfortunate that healing has developed a bit of a shady reputation when linked with faith. Most people associate faith healing with fundamentalist theology, traveling revival preachers, and endless appeals for money. Though faith healing in this form is certainly prominent in the United States, faith has much more to offer to healing than this example might imply.

Most of us use the term faith healing to refer to a purely supernatural event, or a fraudulent imitation of a supernatural event. God acts by divine fiat, bypassing the laws of nature utilized by physicians, and a sick person is instantaneously made well. By the will of the Almighty, "the blind receive their sight, the lame walk, the lepers are cleansed, the deaf hear, the dead are raised," (Luke 7:22).

God can and does heal in this way. Healing was a major focus of Jesus' earthly ministry, and there is no scriptural or theological reason to believe that He refuses to do so now. Jesus also commissioned his disciples to heal. Mark 6:12-13 describes the disciples' activity on their first missionary journey: "So they went out and proclaimed that all should repent. They cast out many demons, and annointed with oil many who were sick and cured them." In the Catholic Church, the annointing of the sick is still practiced today, and many have testified to God's willingness to work through this channel.

Although God can heal supernaturally, He usually chooses not to. Even when Jesus walked the earth, there were many sick people in Palestine who were not miraculously healed. This does not mean that God had no interest in these people, or that He has no interest in those people who are not miraculously healed today. It means that His healing may come through many possible channels, and that He may begin with the mind or spirit before He heals the body.

As discussed in the first chapter, it is a modern habit of mind to assume that the natural world is an autonomous realm, set in motion by God but not directly affected by Him. This is a conception which we have inherited from the eighteenth century Enlightenment. The rationalist philosophers of this period were generally deists, meaning that they believed in God but not necessarily in the Christian revelation. The God of the deists set the world in motion but did not interfere with its regular operation.

Enlightenment thinkers believed that the regularities uncovered by science pointed towards a universe where supernatural events were impossible by definition. This vision of a purely natural reality, whether with a creator God or without, has had an enormous amount of influence ever since. Even many Christians have unconsciously adopted its preconceptions and categories. When applied to healing, this amalgam of Christian and Enlightenment thought classifies any healing which isn't clearly supernatural as a purely biological event, explicable without any reference to God or the spirit.

This is not the vision of Scripture. There is no aspect of creation outside of God's intimate ongoing concern and care. As described in Psalm 104:

> These all look to you to give them their food in due season;
> when you give it to them, they gather it up;
> when you open your hand, they are filled with good things.
> When you hide your face, they are dismayed, when you take away
> their breath, they die and return to their dust.
> When you send forth your spirit, they are created;
> and you renew the face of the ground (Ps. 104:27-30).

If we are healed by an antibiotic, or simply by the passage of time, this is as much an act of God as is the most dramatic miraculous healing. All of creation is God's, and He may choose to act in any number of possible ways. Indeed, Scripture itself teaches that we should take advantage of medical care. "Honor physicians for their services, for the Lord created them; for their gift of healing comes from the Most High," (Sirach 38:1-2).

Even the humble home remedy has its place. St. Paul was certainly no stranger to miraculous healings, and he also had a close association with Luke the physician. Nonetheless, he was willing to pass on a little amateur medical advice to Timothy: "No longer drink only water, but take a little wine for the sake of your stomach and your frequent ailments," (1 Timothy 5:23). God does not require that good advice come only from the mouth of an M.D.

This last assertion is sometimes a stumbling block for those whose thinking is shaped by Enlightenment categories. Many of us assume that the realm of matter is rarely or never influenced by the realm of spirit. Matter is moved only by material influences, in accord with the laws of nature, and so a purely materialist science is the proper tool for understanding it. This, of course, is one of the foundational assumptions of conventional medicine.

The realm of spirit, on the other hand, belongs wholly to God. He may be willing to occasionally cross the divide with a big miracle, but otherwise the two realms remain separate. Any attempt to address the realm of spirit from the other side, the realm of matter, is magic and is therefore forbidden.

This scheme certainly simplifies decision making. There are only two acceptable options when we have a health problem: a conventional M.D., who will stay on his side of the matter/spirit line; or prayer. Anything else is occultism.

Unfortunately, as we have seen, this model is inconsistent with the biblical witness. There is one reality, not two; and there is no part of that reality which is not touched by God. Matter and spirit interpenetrate and influence one another at every point, especially in the human person.

God is transcendent, but He has littered the world with channels and mediators of His grace. He delights in using the humblest substances—bread, wine, water—as vehicles for divinity. He is certainly not contemptuous of matter. He made it, and He loves it.

It is hard to believe that this God would insist that we ignore the presence of spirit in our lives. It is hard to believe that He would want us to treat our bodies as nothing more than complicated mechanisms. It seems far more likely that He would want us to appreciate our essential unity, even if that recognition undercuts our comfortable categories. Even more importantly, it seems the height of folly to place limits on this God and assume that we know how He will act.

It is sobering to remember that Jesus Himself was accused of healing by the power of Satan. He pointed out that "Every kingdom divided against itself is laid waste, and no city or house divided against itself will stand. If Satan casts out Satan, he is divided against himself; how then will his kingdom stand?" (Matthew 12:25-26). We must be very careful of accusing healers of occultism simply because they are unorthodox by the standards of materialist science. If true healing has taken place, then we may assume that God has acted.

Nonetheless, God can heal in spite of a given healing technique as well as through it. We can no more regard anecdotal accounts of success as evidence of God's approval than of scientific validity. Whatever healing discipline we choose to utilize, we must never assume a unique divine sanction simply because we get results.

Medicine, of whatever variety, must be practiced humbly. We can hope that the medicine with which we are treated or with which we treat others will serve as a channel for God's grace, but we must always remember that this is at God's discretion and not ours. No matter how skillful we are, sometimes God's answer is no.

Humility and a sense of our own limits can spare us from several errors. When we first realize that the boundary between matter and spirit is porous, there is a powerful temptation to turn doctors into priests or priests into doctors. The first of these is what often passes for holistic medicine, and the second is the impulse behind more than one Christian sect. Both are equally flawed.

Simply because matter and spirit interact, we cannot assume that knowledge of one gives command of the other. They remain distinct realms, and each must be approached on its own terms. Faith is not a medical instrument to be wielded like a scalpel, and doctors aren't normally qualified to address our spiritual condition.

What we need is a medicine which works on and through natural channels, but which honors the unity of the human person and which is open to the reality of the spiritual. This is generally not true of conventional medicine, which often regards prayer as a last resort to be utilized only after the doctors have failed.

Some of the most revealing material published in conventional medical journals consists of those studies and surveys which attempt to understand the appeal of alternative therapies. The Christian will be startled to discover that these articles frequently include prayer among the ranks of the alternatives (Friedman e1). When physicians admit with dismay that a high percentage of the public utilizes alternatives, this sometimes means only that people pray when they are sick!

Christians, of course, don't regard prayer as an alternative to anything but as a necessary ingredient of everything. There is no part of life that stands apart from our faith, particularly health and illness. We do not want to make the error of King Asa as described in 2 Chronicles 16:12: "In the thirty-ninth year of his reign Asa was diseased in his feet, and his disease became severe; yet even in his disease he did not seek the Lord, but sought help from physicians." Asa's mistake did not lie in consulting doctors, but in refusing to acknowledge God's sovereignty over this part of his life. We too are called to pray; before, during, and after our trip to the doctor.

This doesn't mean that we will refuse to cooperate with our treatment. It is only the uncompromising materialism of conventional medicine that causes its representatives to regard prayer as a competi-tor. Conventional medicine begins with the assumption that the causes of illness can in principle be known with the tools of physical and bio-logical science. If prayer works, then it is an influence that science can-not trace. It becomes a challenge to the all-sufficiency of the biomedical approach.

In contrast, a humble medicine would recognize that we don't have to be able to know everything in order to know something. God is con-stantly at work in the world, and God will always transcend our under-standing, but this does not devalue what we have learned about God's creation. We can use what we know without assuming that our knowl-edge makes us the final arbiters of reality.

Just as we cannot limit the channels through which God may work, we cannot assume that we know the limits of His interest and concern. We assume that God wants to save our souls but is indifferent to our bodies, but instead He wants all of us. We assume that God wants to pull us out of the world, but instead He wants to save the world too. Whenever we try to draw a line to mark out God's circle of concern, we find Him on both sides.

If God will not draw lines, then we shouldn't either. We shouldn't allow ourselves to believe that our illness or our suffering somehow stands alone. When we are ill, we join the multitude of other suffering people for whom Christ died. Indeed, both suffering and God's love extend beyond humanity. As Paul tells us in Romans 8:19-23:

> For the creation waits with eager longing for the revealing of the children of God; for the creation was subjected to futility, not of its own will but by the will of the one who subjected it, in hope that the creation itself will be set free from its bondage to decay and will obtain the freedom of the glory of the children of God. We know that the whole creation has been groaning in labor pains until now; and not only the creation, but we ourselves, who have the first fruits of the Spirit, groan inwardly while we wait for adoption, the redemption of our bodies.

All of creation is wounded, and God intends to heal that wound. That healing began on Calvary and it guaranteed to us by our Lord's sacrifice on the cross. We won't see that healing in its fullness, however, until the end of history.

Until that time comes, we live in a world that has been radically sundered from God by sin. Sin is not just an individual matter. It is corporate in its effects, even trans-human. As Paul put it, "the whole creation has been groaning."

This means that there is a relationship between sickness and sin, but it is not a simple one. Sickness is one of the many evils flowing from creation's great wound. It affects the guilty and the innocent alike. We cannot assume that there is a direct connection between an individual's spiritual health and his or her physical condition. Sometimes sin has an immediate effect on the body of the sinner, but more often we are reminded of the words of the Preacher in Ecclesiastes: "There are righteous people who perish in their righteousness, and there are wicked people who prolong their life in their evil-doing," (Eccl. 7:15).

When we study the lives of the saints, it almost seems as if the righteous are uniquely subject to ill health. Many of the saints have lived with some long-term affliction. Saint Paul complained of his "thorn in the flesh," (2 Cor. 12:7). Saint Ignatius suffered all his life from war wounds. Saint Therese of Lisieux died at an early age of tuberculosis. Sainthood is obviously not a ticket to superior health.

This shouldn't be surprising if we remember the cross. We have the example of our Lord to prove that the innocent often suffer. His example shows us something else, as well: unearned suffering is redemptive. If we are called to bear some illness or discomfort that we don't deserve and don't want, we must remember that our suffering can still have meaning. If we join our afflictions to the cross of Christ, they can participate in that great sacrifice which is remaking the world. We will be able to join with Paul as he proclaims "I am now rejoicing in my sufferings for your sake, and in my flesh I am completing what is lacking in

Christ's afflictions for the sake of his body, that is, the church," (Col. 1:24).

There is nothing wrong with seeking healing, as long as we remember that there is nothing morally wrong with those who are not healed. This will help us to avoid the "health perfectionism" discussed in Chapter Two. We have a deeper commitment than our commitment to health as a goal. We are bound to a Lord who remains always in loving solidarity with the sick and suffering. We must let Him guide us as we begin our exploration of alternative medicine.

4

SORTING THROUGH THE CONFUSION

Alternative medicine would be far easier to deal with if we could just accept or reject it as a whole. This is probably why most people approach it in exactly this way. If we have grown up in a typical American family, then we use conventional medicine for all of our health problems, because that's what our parents did and what everyone else we know does. If conventional medicine has served us well (and most of the time it does), then it is easy to regard alternatives as enclaves of superstition in an otherwise rational modern world.

If, on the other hand, conventional medicine has failed us or a loved one, we may find ourselves in the position described in the first chapter—dissatisfied with the conventional options but uncertain how to proceed with alternatives. The very variety of available possibilities can be baffling. It is all too easy to resort to the shotgun approach to selecting therapies. We use every alternative we can find, in the hope that *something* will prove effective.

This kind of uncritical plunge has its own dangers. Since alternative therapies range from the effective to the ineffective to the actively dangerous, it is possible to throw therapies into the mix that undercut our chances of getting well. We need a more selective set of standards that will allow us to sort useful from useless therapies and avoid any attendant spiritual dangers as well.

This means that we are engaged in a search for truth. We want to find those therapies that are based on truthful beliefs about disease and other, larger issues. We want to avoid those therapies built on a foundation of half truths, misconceptions, or outright falsehoods. It is important to affirm our desire for truth at the outset, because this will help us avoid one of the major spiritual dangers discussed in chapter two—a relativism that makes truth optional depending on personal preference.

In contrast, if we are intent on the truth, then we can be confident that what we find can offer no challenge to our faith. Christianity sustains us precisely because it is true, and truth cannot contradict itself. True faith has nothing to fear from the truth.

Many people find a "search for truth" a more intimidating prospect than a little casual experimentation with herbs or vitamins, but in fact they are the same thing. Any time we sample a little of this or a little of that to see what works, we are engaged in seat-of-the-pants scientific experimentation, and science is a method for uncovering the truth. If we are explicit about our desire to find the truth, then we can examine our standards for success and see if science is the only method that applies.

As Christians, we must establish one standard at the outset and insist that it is not subject to compromise. Our faith comes first. Nothing will be allowed to interfere with or weaken our relationship with the Living God. The Lord our God is a jealous God (Exodus 20:5), and our dependence on Him is absolute.

We have a clear duty to reject any therapy which calls for us to deny our faith. No Christian worthy of the name would disagree with this. Unfortunately, our choice is rarely this clear cut. While there are healing practices associated with certain cults that might lead us to deny our Christian commitment, most people will never be faced with this kind of ordeal. (If you do find yourself entangled with this kind of cult, I would encourage you to seek help as quickly as possible from a trusted family member or friend *outside* the cult.) Instead, most of us will be faced with far more ambiguous choices.

We may be offered training in a meditative technique or mind-body method that doesn't explicitly deny anything we believe but which clearly comes from another religious tradition. We may meet a proponent or practitioner of a given therapy who also proselytizes for a non-Christian faith. We may discover re-interpretations of Christianity that are so far removed from mainstream beliefs that we wonder if they are orthodox. What do we do in these cases? Do they constitute a denial of our faith?

It should be said that not all of these hypothetical cases are clearly wrong, and one can imagine thoughtful, careful Christians going forward under these kinds of circumstances. For instance, I would be comfortable receiving acupuncture from someone who practiced Buddhism or Taoism in their personal life. I see no more reason to object to this than I would to receiving treatment from a Jewish dentist. If a therapy does not depend on spiritual mechanisms, then the faith commitments of the practitioner and the patient are irrelevant.

Just as these instances seem clearly safe, there are others that are clearly unsafe. If a given practice is an occult or religious ritual that attempts to draw upon the powers of gods or spirits other than the God of Abraham, Isaac, and Jacob, then it is unacceptable to Christians whether it is called alternative medicine or not. For instance, shamanism has become quite popular in some alternative circles. It is not uncommon for holistic healing events to include exercises in which the participants attempt to contact their "spirit guide" or "power animal". No Christian should engage in these practices.

In the middle are practices which may have had their origins in other religious traditions, but which are now stripped of religious content and presented in secular terms as techniques for relaxation or healing. There are a variety of meditative techniques and breath control regimens that began centuries ago as paths to enlightenment which are now taught as ways to handle the stress of modern life. With these techniques no simple answer is possible. The acceptability of a given practice may vary from individual to individual, depending upon circumstances, motivation, and strength of faith.

I am certain that there are many Christians who can use these practices safely. If your heart is wholly focused on the love of God, then anything which stills the mind can deepen your prayer life. "To the pure all things are pure," (Titus 1:15). We should not erect legalistic barriers to the wisdom of other faiths.

At the same time, I think some caution is warranted. Very few of us are saints. Our devotion to God is real, but if we are honest we must admit that it is sometimes weak. We are sometimes drawn to goals that are inconsistent with our faith. If this is the state of our spiritual development, then we need to be careful that these meditative practices don't become an alternative to prayer.

They offer an enticing set of rewards. The proponents of these techniques promise us peace of mind through the mastery of ourselves. If this peace of mind is not rooted in the Lord, then it is ultimately illusory. There is no true peace outside of Christ.

There is an alternative for those of us who might be troubled by these concerns. Rather than rely on practices about which we are uncertain, we can draw on the riches of our own tradition. Christianity offers a wealth of meditative, centering prayers which can both quiet our minds and turn our hearts to God. Those of us who are Catholic have usually grown up with the rosary. When prayed with full attention the rosary is one of Christendom's most profound and glorious prayers. The Eastern Orthodox have the Jesus Prayer, consisting of the repetition of "Lord Jesus Christ, Son of God, have mercy on me," in union with the breath. For those who are advanced students of Christian mysticism, the works of St. Theresa of Avila and St. John of the Cross offer a great deal.

Lately, even the most prominent advocates of secularized meditation have begun to acknowledge that prayer is not only more spiritually sound, but also more conducive to health benefits than meditation practiced solely for relaxation. Herbert Benson of Harvard Medical

School originated the phrase "the relaxation response" to describe the physiological changes which can be produced by meditative practices. His book by that name was one of the earliest and most influential attempts to introduce meditation to the American mainstream. He now recommends that the meditator focus on a prayer or some other phrase with religious meaning for that person in order to achieve the greatest possible benefits (Benson 60-67). Christian prayer is on the alternative cutting edge!

Christianity also offers superior substitutes for the various "energy healing" therapies like Reiki or Therapeutic Touch. These therapies all use some variation of the laying on of hands in order to transmit a putative healing energy to the patient. Almost all of the various Christian traditions practice some form of healing, although it is probably most common among Pentecostals and Roman Catholics. Though some Catholics may be surprised by this statement, the Church has moved to restore the sacrament once known as the Last Rites to the position it held in the early Church as the Anointing of the Sick. This sacrament is available to any Catholic who is seriously ill, not just the dying.

Relying on Christian healing will protect us from some theological errors that seem particularly common among practitioners of energy therapies. These practitioners frequently draw parallels between the healing energy they believe they are manipulating and the Holy Spirit (Maxwell 96-99). Since the Holy Spirit is somewhat mysterious to most Christians, these parallels have a superficial plausibility.

Unfortunately, the Holy Spirit is not a force or energy that can be manipulated at our pleasure. He is a person, the third member of the Trinity, and is as deserving of our worship as the other members of the Godhead. If we believe that we can control the grace of His healing power through a technique, like flipping a light switch, then we have strayed into occultism. We are at God's disposal, not vice versa.

Though Christian healing sometimes resembles the energy therapies in its outward forms, there is a crucial difference. Christian healing is always a prayer, a humble request rather than a command. The advantage of staying within our tradition is that it helps us to remember this.

Despite the holistic perspective of the alternative community, most alternative therapies are more purely medical than spiritual in orientation. There is no reason to assume that a conflict with the conventional biomedical establishment will inevitably lead to a conflict with Christianity. When there is no conflict with our faith, we must use a new set of criteria to evaluate these therapies. Our primary concerns are effectiveness and safety. Some of the most powerful tools for uncovering the truth when we are faced with this kind of question are those developed by modern science.

Science functions by isolating the smallest possible part of a problem, holding everything else steady, and then experimentally manipulating the isolated element. By breaking complex problems into smaller elements, scientific investigation is able to build a picture of the whole through the painstaking analysis of the parts. The careful control of as many variable elements in the environment as possible allows a clear picture to emerge of the relationship between the experimental manipulation and the results obtained. In contrast to the world outside the laboratory, where a thousand subtle influences may be impacting on the most trivial event, the clean and unambiguous experiments of science can uncover cause and effect relationships with a high degree of assurance.

Scientific investigation in medicine has some unique problems, however. Though animal experiments can provide useful information, ultimately they cannot provide definitive conclusions about the value of medical interventions intended for human beings. Only human experiments can do that. Unfortunately, human beings make poor experimental animals.

We are too complicated to allow the easy isolation of a variable in an experimental setting. We come equipped with beliefs and expectations which alter our response to therapeutic interventions. A therapy which has no real physiological impact may produce a beneficial effect if we think it will. This, of course, is the famous placebo effect.

In addition, we are too good at communicating with one another, even if we don't intend to. An investigator can communicate his expectations about the value of a therapy to the subjects of a trial intended to establish that value. This can take place through completely nonverbal, unconscious channels. As a result, the investigator can produce the placebo effect in his subjects if his own belief in the therapy is strong.

The medical research community has several ways of dealing with these difficulties. In order to correct for the effect of the subjects' expectations, some of the subjects can be given an inactive medication, a sugar pill that resembles the real drug in every way except for the presence of the active ingredient. The investigators can then measure the difference between the two groups to isolate the effect of the drug from the effect of the patients' belief in it. An experiment designed in this way is called a placebo-controlled trial.

To ensure that the investigators themselves do not communicate their expectations to the people receiving the real drug, the identity of these people is frequently concealed from the investigators until the trial is completed. If an experiment has this added layer of security, then it is considered double-blind, because neither the scientists nor the subjects know who is receiving the real intervention. A double-blind placebo-controlled trial is considered the most authoritative kind of medical experiment, because the greatest possible care has been taken to isolate the effect of the therapy being tested from possible confounding factors.

If the medical literature contains several double-blind placebo-controlled trials evaluating a therapy we are interested in, this is the best possible kind of evidence. These trials need to have survived the process of peer review by other scientists both before and after publication, and the trials should be in general agreement with one another, but if both these hurdles have been crossed then we can regard the information provided by the trials as reasonably sound. It is still possible for the conclusions drawn from the trials to be incorrect if there is a hidden variable affecting the results, if the results have been improperly analyzed, or if outright fraud has occurred, but this is highly unlikely if the trials were well designed. In general double-blind placebo-controlled trials provide the most reliable medical information available.

It is important to establish this, because there is much sniping by the alternative community at the ideal of the controlled trial, for both good and bad reasons. The most prominent bad reason is one that conventional physicians love to point out—some, though not all, alternative therapies cannot survive the degree of scrutiny implied by the controlled trial. When examined closely they just don't work.

Though this is sometimes true, there are also good reasons to remain aware of the limitations of the controlled trial. Controlled trials depend upon standardizing both the experimental population and the treatment being studied as much as possible. This works well for conventional therapies, where standardized treatments for specific diseases are the norm. Many alternative therapies are much more focused on the patient than the disease. A patient's unique individual characteristics may well determine treatment rather than the disease category the patient has been assigned to by Western medicine. Traditional Chinese medicine, for instance, analyzes patients in terms wholly foreign to the West. Two patients who both have the disease "rheumatoid arthritis" in Western terms may receive entirely different treatments. This makes the design of a controlled trial acceptable to both the traditional practitioner and the Western scientist difficult.

It is not, however, impossible, despite the complaints of many alternative practitioners. A trial can be constructed in which the patient population is standardized by both the conventional diagnosis and the alternative category and treatment. In the example given above, a trial could be run using only those rheumatoid arthritis patients with deficient kidney yin in Chinese terms, so that the Chinese therapy could be standardized. Another possibility is to allow the alternative practitioners to treat any given patient as they see fit. Though this adds a layer of complexity that would make it virtually impossible to test every detail and every available therapy in a given alternative system, enough trials could be run to establish whether the system taken as a whole has any power to affect illness. Though it is unlikely that each of the hundreds of possible homeopathic remedies will be tested in double-blind controlled trials, enough trials can be run to allow us to state with some assurance whether or not the dilute remedies used by homeopathy are capable of activity.

A more difficult problem is that not all alternative therapies lend themselves to blinding. It is hard to see how a chiropractor could give a sham adjustment without being aware that he was doing so, or how an acupuncturist could be induced to needle points without knowing whether they are correct or not. In the case of chiropractic, it is likely that even the patient could easily tell the difference between a real and a placebo adjustment.

Sympathetic researchers who have thought about this problem have proposed "outcomes-based" research as a solution. Outcomes-based studies observe the clinical results obtained when two otherwise comparable groups are treated with two different therapies. A standard therapy of known effectiveness takes the place of a placebo. Much of the research funded by the new Office of Alternative Medicine in the National Institutes of Health follows this model.

This is not a perfect solution. The lack of blinding does allow more room for bias to operate. Nonetheless, in some cases, this is the best that can be done. It is unfair for conventional physicians to criticize therapies subject to these constraints in experimental design because they haven't met the standard of the double-blind placebo-controlled trial. A therapy may be quite effective even though its nature prevents us from demonstrating that effectiveness with the perfect air-tight experiment.

A final problem with double-blind controlled trials is that they are expensive and difficult to run. This means that funding authorities tend to reserve these trials for situations where there is a high degree of scientific consensus about the anticipated outcome, or at a minimum, situations where any controversy provides a limited number of clear, easily distinguished ways of understanding the data. Controlled trials are run to evaluate mainstream therapies that are close to widespread application. Off the wall ideas will not be funded.

By definition, this tends to exclude most alternatives. Advocates of alternative therapies are caught between a rock and a hard place, because they are condemned for failing to provide the kind of evidence that would satisfy conventional physicians while at the same time they are excluded from most of the institutional funding sources that would allow them to conduct this kind of research. Any investigator with too much interest in an alternative therapy will receive well-intentioned hints from colleagues or mentors that such an interest may impact adversely on one's career.

The real problem is not the controlled trial, or any of the other tools of science. The real problem is the culture of science. Science has developed a set of tools of enormous power, but they are not, indeed cannot, be applied to every possible problem. Scientists choose those areas for investigation that they believe will be most fruitful. This selection process depends on the pre-existing beliefs and biases of the scientists doing the choosing.

Unfortunately, as discussed in chapter one, there is an enormously powerful bias towards materialism in the culture of science. Alternative therapies in general have a vitalist orientation, which tends to exclude them from serious scientific examination at the outset. Even when institutional science does consider alternatives, it is almost always with the stated or unstated goal of uncovering the *real* mechanism of action. This, of course, is assumed to be either the placebo effect or some chemical or mechanical process. Genuine anomalies which resist conventional explanations are dismissed or ignored.

This puts us in a difficult position if we are seeking information about these therapies. If good controlled trials exist, we should seek them out and pay attention to their findings. All too often, however, these trials either don't exist or are insufficiently rigorous to allow us to make a decision. This may not be because of any deficiency in the therapy but simply because it is too far removed from the perspective of mainstream scientists to attract their attention. What do we do then?

If the full focus of institutional science has not been directed toward a therapy we find interesting, then we are forced to accept a lower standard of proof. We have to know this going in, and be willing to accept that good ideas, even good ideas which seem to make sense of the available data, are frequently wrong. It is the great and largely unique achievement of science to have developed a method for discarding good ideas which are unfortunately untrue. If we are unwilling to take a chance on ideas which have not passed through this screening process, then we should stick with conventional medicine. Though even conventional medicine does not apply the scientific method with perfect consistency, conventional therapies are far more likely to have survived this kind of examination than unconventional therapies.

This doesn't mean that unconventional therapies don't work. It simply means that we don't know whether they work or not with the same degree of assurance that we can have regarding conventional medicine. Nonetheless, we can assemble information from various sources that will allow us to make a tentative decision.

We should pay attention to the expert opinions offered by physicians and scientists, but we should also be aware of the limitations of those opinions. The mind of an expert, steeped in the minutiae of his or her discipline, can sometimes produce an intuitive assessment of astonishing accuracy, but they can also be wrong. We need to watch for the "well, that's just stupid" objection to alternative perspectives. If this is not based on solid experimental evidence, then it is just another example of the materialist bias of the scientific community.

In a similar vein are the "How to Spot a Quack" checklists frequently distributed by consumer oriented health organizations. There is such a thing as real quackery, but these checklists rarely serve to distinguish it from other alternative therapies. Many of the standards proposed tend to exclude any therapy which is not a part of the conventional medical establishment.

For instance, these checklists frequently list among the characteristics of quacks the belief that there is an organized conspiracy by the institutions of regular medicine to suppress their revolutionary therapy. It is one of the quirks of the alternative community that this belief is held by a very large number, probably a majority, of people working with alternative therapies. Part of this is the reflexive anti-establishment paranoia inherited from the counter-culture.

Part of it, however, is the well established historical fact that organized medicine has engaged in several attempts to destroy medical alternatives that seemed particularly threatening. Whether you regard this as consumer protection or a conspiracy depends on which side of the fence you are standing on. The A.M.A., for instance, was founded in the nineteenth century to protect "scientific" medicine (which at that time consisted largely of bleeding, purging, and the administration of toxic drugs made from heavy metals) from the threat posed by homeopathy. In the twentieth century the federal courts have held that the A.M.A. did in fact engage in a criminal conspiracy to destroy chiropractic. Some skepticism about the open minded goodwill of regular medicine does seem warranted.

So in many ways we are on our own. We cannot rely on the usual voices of authority to provide us with the kind of dispassionate but religiously informed judgement that we seek. Neither can we expect a careful, rational assessment from the advocates of alternative therapies, particularly if we hope for an assessment that is sympathetic to Christian sensibilities. When we seek an expert opinion, we find that the loudest voices we hear stand for either an aggressive skepticism which elevates Science to the position of a god, or a vaguely New Age wooly mindedness that is willing to let almost anything be elevated to divine status. Real rationality and the real God are ignored in this debate.

Whenever we attempt to evaluate an unconventional therapy we should begin from the perspective of faith. We should ask God for the gift of discernment and we should stay in prayer as we attempt to make medical decisions. Then we can begin sifting the evidence. This should almost always begin with a trip to the library.

We are looking for two kinds of literature. The first are solid controlled studies in the biomedical literature which evaluate the therapy we are interested in. Ideally these studies would be large, randomized so that the control group and the intervention group are as equivalent as possible, placebo-controlled, double-blind, and if possible repeated several times by different investigators. A good librarian can help us discover if these studies exist.

After we have surveyed the biomedical literature we can move on to the second type of writing—books and articles by advocates of the therapy. We want to ensure that the therapy does not involve the worship of gods other than our own, or occult practices in which the will is harnessed by ritual or concentration exercises to influence the world through paranormal channels. If a therapy can pass these hurdles, then we can begin examining the history of the therapy and the clinical experience accumulated by its practitioners.

As we read this literature, we must always remain aware of the power of the placebo effect. This is why stories of individual cases, no matter how dramatic they may seem, are almost worthless as evidence. We should be as critical of anecdotal evidence as the most tough minded physician.

We are looking for a long history of clinical success, replicated by many practitioners. If no one has duplicated the results achieved by a single person, then we have no way of knowing if they *could* be duplicated. One person can easily be deceived, or deceitful. A hundred people can be too, but it is less likely. If thousands of people, over many years or centuries, report the same results, then something of interest is probably present.

We should also read with an eye to seeing if the ideas underlying a therapy make sense. Common sense and intuition can be deceived, so they aren't perfect guides. Nonetheless, if something rings an alarm bell in our minds, we should heed that warning.

One way of assessing the inherent reasonableness of a practice or a practitioner is to see if they accept and acknowledge the world's legitimate complexity. Human health and illness are complicated processes. There is no single unitary cause of disease, whether it be germs, bad genes, spinal subluxation, bad diet, or bad thinking. Anyone who argues that all disease can be traced back to some single central cause has so oversimplified the problem that one must doubt their ability to fix it. Diseases have many causes, and any one disease may have several distinct but mutually interacting causes. It may be necessary to approach an illness on several levels to achieve real healing.

And we must always remember that the health of our bodies is not the highest good. The pursuit of perfect health can lead to dangerous self absorption. All things must be brought back to God.

If we keep these general principles in mind, then the jungle of alternative therapies needn't seem so forbidding. We can begin to clear away the confusion, examining specific individual therapies. If we bring both our reason and our faith to bear, then we can discover what they may have to offer us.

5

DIET

Almost all Americans have had the experience of modifying their diet to achieve some health goal. Though many of the hazards we face in life are beyond our ability to control, we can, at least in the short term, decide what we are going to put in our mouths. It seems intuitively satisfying that diet would have a profound effect on our health, and most of us accept this as an article of faith. We do argue vigorously about exactly how our diet should be changed.

Conventional physicians generally agree that a healthy diet has less fat, less salt, and more fruits and vegetables than the standard American diet, but even they disagree about the details. Fat should be cut to 30%, 20%, or 10% of calories. Oat bran does or does not prevent heart disease. Alcoholic beverages are or are not good for you, and if they are, then it must be red wine, or not. Fat should be polyunsaturated, or monounsaturated. Beta carotene does or does not prevent cancer.

Given this lack of consensus, it is not surprising that there are a number of alternative diet schemes competing with conventional advice for the consumer's attention. Here there is even more diversity. Some systems are built around the idea that grain should be the primary constituent of the diet, since it is the staple food of nonindustrialized peasant peoples around the world. Others argue that grain is the source of all our ills, since it was relatively unknown to our hunter-gatherer ancestors and only became a large part of the human diet with the invention of agriculture. Similar disagreements rage about the value of meat, dairy products, and fruit. Indeed, all of the primary macronutrients, meaning protein, carbohydrates, and fats, have been indicted by one group or another as a cause of human disease. If one eliminated all foods condemned as unhealthy, there would be nothing left to eat at all.

Nonetheless, hope springs eternal, so we continue to tinker with our diets in the hope of achieving youth, beauty, and health. The American obsession with weight loss, combined with the generally unsatisfactory nature of all the available treatments for obesity, results in a constant demand for new diet schemes. They are so common that they hardly seem unusual, yet they are probably the most common way that people first step beyond conventional medical authority. In this sense, they are "gateways" to more sweeping alternative perspectives.

Theologically, there is little to choose between them. Christian faith does not require any particular style of eating, and mainstream Christianity has generally rejected the idea that one diet is more moral than another, assuming, of course, that gluttony is not involved. As Jesus said in Matthew 15: 10-11, "Listen and understand: it is not what goes into the mouth that defiles a person, but it is what comes out of the mouth that defiles."

This was a very controversial issue in the early Church. Many of the first Christians were converts from Judaism, and initially the relationship between the two faiths was not clear. Most of the new Jewish Christians rightfully regarded Christianity as the fulfillment of God's promises to the Jews, rather than a new religion. These Christians thought of themselves as Jews, still bound to observe the Law with all its dietary regulations. When Gentiles entered the Church, it was often assumed that these Gentile converts would need to become Jews in order to become Christians. This would include circumcision and observance of the dietary rules.

On the other side of this issue was Saint Paul, who preached that the Gospel had set all people free from the ritual demands of the Jewish Law. The issue was settled at the Council of Jerusalem recorded in Acts

15. Paul gathered with the other apostles and the elders of the Church to settle the status of the Gentile converts and the role of the Law.

The solution, as expressed by James in Acts 15: 19-20, was something of a compromise. Most of the demands of the Law were lifted, and converts were asked to avoid only the most obvious and public violations of the Law. They were to "abstain only from things polluted by idols and from fornication and from whatever has been strangled and from blood," (Acts 15: 20).

It seems likely that this compromise was intended to avoid scandalizing Jewish Christians so as to prevent a public split. Paul discusses the obligation to avoid shocking those who are weak in faith in 1 Corinthians 8. He makes it plain that there is no objective sin involved in eating meat sacrificed to idols. "Food will not bring us close to God. We are no worse off if we do not eat, and no better off if we do," (1 Cor. 8: 8). Still, we may sin by unnecessarily confusing those who do not understand this and thereby tempting them to disobey their own consciences. "But take care that this liberty of yours does not become a stumbling block to the weak. For if others see you, who possess knowledge, eating in the temple of an idol, might they not, since their conscience is weak, be encouraged to the point of eating food sacrificed to idols? So by your knowledge those weak believers for whom Christ died are destroyed," (1 Cor. 8: 9-11).

Once the Church had developed its own public identity, even these minimal concessions to Jewish dietary law were largely forgotten. To a degree this may have been because they were no longer necessary. As the ancient world became increasingly Christianized, pagan temples were no longer the primary sites for butchering meat. Dietary regulations became purely devotional practices, limited to specific days and times. The rationale for a Christian vegetarianism had always been limited and contingent, and now it disappeared altogether. As Paul wrote in Romans 14: 17, "For the kingdom of God is not food and drink but righteousness and peace and joy in the Holy Spirit."

Since there is essentially no evidence for a "Christian diet" in the New Testament, defenders of the concept frequently turn to the Old Testament for scriptural justification. Common proof texts offered as a religious defense of vegetarianism include Genesis 1: 29-30 and Daniel 1: 12-16. Neither of these passages can support the arguments vegetarians have attempted to build on them.

In Genesis 1: 29-30, God gives every green plant for food to everything that has the breath of life. This is superficially convincing, until one notes that in Genesis 9: 2-4 God alters his provision for humankind. "Every moving thing that lives shall be food for you; and just as I gave you the green plants, I give you everything," (Gen. 9: 3). If we give up flesh foods for moral reasons, we are being more scrupulous than God. That hardly seems reasonable.

Daniel 1: 12-16 takes place during the Babylonian captivity, when Israel was ruled by Babylon and many of the people were forcibly removed from their homes to live in the land of their conqueror. Daniel and his companions, usually known by the Babylonian names Shadrach, Meshach, and Abednego, were young nobles of the tribe of Judah. They were taken by force to the palace of King Nebuchadnezzar, where they were to be taught Babylonian culture.

This is the context for the quiet battle over food depicted in the passage. The royal rations offered to Daniel and his friends were not acceptable by the standards of Jewish dietary law, no matter how sumptuous they were to the palate. In Daniel 1: 8 the young aristocrat affirms that he will live by God's law, no matter how difficult that might be. "But Daniel resolved that he would not defile himself with the royal ration of food and wine."

This resolve is the source of Daniel's request to live on a vegetarian diet, depicted in Daniel 1: 12-16. "'Please test your servants for ten days. Let us be given vegetables to eat and water to drink. You can then compare our appearance with the appearance of the young men who eat the royal rations, and deal with your servants according to what you observe.' So he (the palace master) agreed to this proposal and tested them for ten days. At the end of the ten days it was observed that they appeared better and fatter than all the young men who had been eating the royal rations. So the guard continued to withdraw their royal rations and the wine they were to drink, and gave them vegetables."

Daniel and his friends choose vegetables, not because they are healthier, but because they are the only reliably kosher foods they can obtain. Their good health on this diet is because of God's miraculous provision for those who live by His law even under adverse circumstances. The young men who eat the royal rations have abandoned the covenant, and they suffer accordingly. The vegetarian diet in this passage is a response to specific circumstances, not a general prescription for health.

One scriptural argument for dietary reform does hold up. As Paul tells us in 1 Corinthians 6: 19, our body is a temple of the Holy Spirit. We each have an obligation to take care of our body. It is indeed sacred.

This scriptural warrant does not dictate any particular kind of diet, as long as it is moderate and healthy. We still need to determine exactly what a healthy diet is. This is a scientific question, and should be approached with the tools of science discussed in the previous chapter.

We are faced with an immediate problem. We know that the most authoritative kind of evidence is provided by the double-blind controlled trial. Neither the experimenters nor the subjects should know who has received the therapeutic intervention. This is almost impossible to arrange when the intervention is a change in diet. People almost always know what they are eating, unless they are willing to check themselves into a hospital and receive tube feedings. Since some diet changes aren't believed to affect health risks until they have been practiced for months or years, a true blinded trial becomes almost inconceivable.

Unblinded trials are subject to all the vagaries of expectation and the placebo effect. In addition, compliance is always an issue with diet changes. As those of us who have tried to stick to a diet know, it's hard to be good. It's also embarrassing to admit that you've cheated, so people don't always own up to their dietary sins, especially if they are talking to an authority figure like a doctor or a scientist. Unless investigators are willing to lock their subjects up or follow them day and night, they can never be certain of the accuracy of their data.

Because of these problems, there are almost no trials examining the impact of diet on health that can meet even the most minimal standards of evidence required for most other kinds of interventions. This is true for even the most mainstream, conservative recommendations. Almost all of what we think we know about diet has been assembled from another kind of evidence—epidemiological associations.

Epidemiology is the study of associations between factors in the environment and health or disease. The object is to figure out which things in the environment vary in the same way as the disease being studied. For instance, different countries have different rates of heart disease. Diet also varies from country to country. If epidemiologists can find an aspect of diet that mirrors the changes in the rate of heart disease, then there may be a causal relationship between the two. The variation in diet may be causing the variation in coronary artery disease.

This is the way dietary fat was indicted as the chief cause of vascular disease. Scientists began building their case with Ancel Keys' classic Seven Countries Study (Keys et al. 1-392), which showed that heart disease rose as the saturated fat content of a country's typical diet rose. Within the United States, a large study of the population of Framingham, Massachusetts had shown the importance of blood cholesterol levels as a risk factor for heart disease (Kahn and Dawber 611-620). Much lab work had convinced scientists that saturated fat was the chief dietary variable capable of affecting cholesterol levels. It seemed like all the pieces were in place.

This is a very truncated sketch of the research which served to convince most of the scientific community of the role played by fat in the genesis of heart disease. It does, however, serve to show the nature of the evidence which has been assembled. It consists, for the most part, of suggestive associations linked by a chain of reasoning. The perfect intervention trial has not, indeed cannot, be done. Some dietary intervention trials have been attempted, but they have not produced impressive results (Moore 194; Corr 18-22). Not one of the trials has produced clear, unambiguous evidence that mortality can be lowered and life extended by altering diet. No matter how well the pieces seem to fit together, epidemiology can never offer the certainty of a good clinical trial, and the clinical trials simply do not exist to support the dietary recommendations we receive from every quarter.

Most people find this a startling assertion. It is worth taking a closer look at one of the most widely publicized trials to see why the evidence it offers is not as strong as most of us assume. The experiment was called The Lifestyle Heart Trial, and it was published in the prestigious journal The Lancet in 1990. The chief investigator was Dr. Dean Ornish, and he parlayed the success of his experiment into widespread celebrity and a series of best-selling books.

Ornish's achievement was to provide the first scientifically acceptable evidence that the artery blocking disease process of atherosclerosis could be reversed by lifestyle changes alone, without drugs or surgery. This is a remarkable achievement, one not to be minimized. Ornish has established that reversal is possible, and until he did it, there was great skepticism about whether it could be done at all.

At the same time, we don't know *how* Ornish accomplished this with his patients. His program is a complex one, involving an extremely low fat vegetarian diet, yoga, walking, meditation, and group support. Any or all of these elements might be the active component. We don't know until additional trials test each of the elements separately and in combination. Media reporting on Ornish's experiment has tended to assume that the diet is the most important part of the program, but this is an assumption only. We just don't know.

We also don't know if the relatively modest degree of reversal which Ornish has demonstrated will translate into a significant difference in mortality. Ornish's experimental group began with twenty eight members and is now down to twenty (Ornish 2001-2007). It is just too small to show a clear mortality difference with the control group. The Ornish program is not a panacea. One member of the lifestyle intervention group has already died of heart disease while on the program (Gerber 62-66). The precise difference in mortality which could be expected if the experimental group and the control group consisted of a few thousand rather than a few dozen people remains to be determined.

Finally, not only did Ornish fail to guard against the possibility of a placebo effect, it almost seems as though he designed his trial to produce such an effect. The experimental group met together on a regular basis to encourage one another and keep each other's motivation up. These meetings were chaired by Ornish himself, who regularly exhorted the group with virtual sermons on the significance of their efforts. All of this seems calculated to produce the kind of expectation and excitement which is known to trigger potent placebo responses whether the experimental intervention has any activity or not.

In short Dean Ornish has demonstrated that a complex, time and labor intensive program of lifestyle modification can produce some reversal of coronary atherosclerosis. He has not demonstrated that any single element of his program could produce the same results, or even that the program as a whole could produce results if it was taken out of its original context and replicated elsewhere without the emotional support provided by his direct involvement. He has not demonstrated that his program can lengthen life. And, in contrast to the most common misconception about his results, Dean Ornish most certainly has not demonstrated that heart disease can be cured by an extremely low fat diet. His results do not qualify as a cure and they cannot be attributed to diet alone.

Any of the other high profile experiments concerning diet and health could be analyzed in this same fashion. Usually the evidence they provide is even less satisfying than that offered by Ornish. Decision making on the basis of these results is complicated by the generally low quality of media reporting about health and medicine. Few of us have access to major university research libraries, so normally we will not be reading these studies in the scientific journals that published them. We will be reading a reporter's summary in a newspaper or magazine. Unfortunately, reporters rarely emphasize or even mention the differences between different kinds of research. They tend to treat all studies as the final word on a subject, whether they are preliminary epidemiological investigations or true blinded clinical trials.

This lack of discernment by the media is largely responsible for the common perception that the dietary advice offered by scientists changes so frequently as to be worthless. Members of the scientific community understand that no single study is ever conclusive. Understanding is achieved gradually, by the accumulation and interpretation of a large body of research. All research must be interpreted carefully, with close attention to possible confounding factors and the details of study design. Conclusions are limited and tentative.

None of this uncertainty is communicated by the media. We need to look past the nutritional fad of the moment, whether it is conventional or alternative, to take a deeper look at diet, health, and how we make decisions about them. Since we must eat, we will make decisions about diet one way or another regardless of the lack of conclusive evidence.

This is an important point. Circumstances sometimes force us to make decisions even when a degree of uncertainty remains about our options. Conventional physicians implicitly acknowledge this when they make dietary recommendations based on the imperfect evidence that we currently have. It is not certain that lowering dietary fat will reduce heart disease, but physicians advise us to do so because the theory is plausible and the intervention itself is conservative and carries little risk.

We can use this kind of decision making to evaluate other, less mainstream options. As Christians, not bound to the pure materialism of current science, our assessment of plausibility may differ significantly from that of the conventionally minded scientists who dominate media reporting about alternative medicine. Once we have allowed ourselves to consider options outside the range of "official" acceptability, we will find that many alternatives actually expose us to less risk than conventional therapies. This applies to both dietary and nondietary approaches.

When we are evaluating dietary approaches, we should always return to the scriptural evidence. God has given us everything for food (Gen. 9: 3). Though we should practice moderation at all times, avoiding drunkenness and gluttony, there are no foods prohibited to us. As Sirach teaches, "Do not deprive yourself of a day's enjoyment; do not let your share of desired good pass by you," (Sirach 14: 14). The enjoyment of food is one of God's gifts to us.

Human beings seem to thrive on a variety of diets. Thomas Moore has pointed out that there is little consistency among the diets of the nations with the world's most long lived populations (Moore 27). The difference between the average life expectancy in Japan, with its exceptionally low fat diet, and Switzerland, with its very high fat diet, is one year for men. For women, there is no difference in life expectancy at all (Reddy 465, 889). Surveys of centenarians have actually shown that they tend to eat *more* fat than those a few decades younger (Houston et al. 5-23).

What does vary between nations are the rates of various diseases. One way to put this is that you can't lengthen your life by altering your diet, but you can pick what you want to die from. For most of us, current understanding of the causes of these varying disease rates is probably too limited to make this a very practical possibility. If, however, an individual already has a disease or a clear susceptibility to a disease, epidemiological associations do provide clues to low risk ways to treat a given condition. A middle aged American man with high cholesterol and a family history of early death from heart disease may find it very interesting that the Japanese diet seems to give them some protection from this condition, regardless of the other diseases they suffer from.

This means that there is no such thing as a single perfect diet which can be prescribed for everyone. Each of us has our own set of weaknesses and susceptibilities which should be considered when we attempt to improve our diet. Alternative dietary approaches are frequently better at appreciating these individual differences.

As an example, hypoglycemia has been a favorite diagnosis in the alternative community for many years. Thousands of people have insisted that refined sugar in foods propels their blood sugar into an unstable roller coaster ride, varying wildly between high and low values and producing moodiness and depression. These self-proclaimed hypoglycemics have maintained that a high protein, low sugar diet with frequent small meals can control their condition and make them feel better.

The response of conventional physicians was, and is, derisive. Studies showed that the blood sugar of self-diagnosed hypoglycemics was no more unstable than that of most normal people. Doctors authoritatively announced that hypoglycemia was a fad diagnosis and that true hypoglycemia was an extremely rare condition. Within the medical community, it was generally assumed that hypoglycemics were in fact neurotics, more in need of psychiatric care than anything else.

Within the last few years, a quiet change began to take place in the conventional understanding of the impact of dietary carbohydrates like sugar. First, Richard and Judith Wurtman showed that carbohydrates were capable of altering the balance of neurotransmitters in the brain by altering the absorption of the amino acids from which they are built (Wurtman et al. 520-528). Gerald Reaven began to accumulate evidence that a sensitivity to carbohydrates (now renamed insulin insensitivity or "Syndrome X") might be a serious risk factor for heart disease in some people (Reaven 948-952). Finally, psychiatric research began to reveal that there might be a small class of sugar sensitive people who would react to excess dietary sugar with moodiness and depression

(Christensen 136-141) Interestingly, the same popular articles which reported the new research often asserted with equal authority the conventional wisdom that hypoglycemics were deluded, as though the new findings had no relationship to the experiences of those hypoglycemics!

The whole episode revealed the worst in both the alternative and the conventional camps. Members of the alternative community were the first to notice a real relationship. Dietary sugar made some people feel bad, and they improved when the sugar was cleaned out of their diet. Having noticed this, they immediately leaped to the conclusion that the understood the mechanism, and then appropriated a piece of standard medical terminology to describe it. The revealed truth about hypoglycemia was then trumpeted to the public through paperback books and popular health magazines. Anyone who disagreed was assumed to be a part of a vast conspiracy of M.D.'s to suppress the truth about the real cause of (by now) most human illness.

The medical community was no more impressive. Having failed to notice the relationship between sugar and mood, physicians in general were not interested in having a promising line of research suggested by laypeople. A few experiments were conducted, but they were designed to test the alternative explanation of the relationship, not the relationship itself. In other words, instead of looking to see if some people reacted to sugar by becoming depressed, researchers fed hypoglycemics sugar and then tested their blood glucose. When this fell within normal values, the whole idea of hypoglycemia was ridiculed. The idea that sugar sensitivity might have another mechanism of action, such as an effect on neurotransmitter balance, seems not to have occurred to anyone.

The alternative community was too quick to leap to the conclusion that they had discovered a panacea. When this was challenged, alternative thinkers reacted with a degree of defensive paranoia and even anti-intellectualism. The medical community showed itself to be highly insular and largely uninterested in ideas or observations coming from anyone without an M.D. or a Ph.D. When they did deign to test the hypoglycemia hypothesis, physicians clearly trusted the results of lab tests more than the reports of the suffering individuals. If blood glucose values were normal, then hypoglycemics were presumed to be psychiatric patients.

A similar process may be taking place in some current dietary controversies. Many holistic practitioners today love to diagnose multiple food allergies in their patients. They use a variety of scientific and pseudo-scientific techniques to uncover these allergies, and their patients end up avoiding long lists of foods to treat conditions which regular medicine does not link to diet.

The response of conventional physicians has been to point out that these sensitivities, if they exist, do not meet the technical definition of a true allergy. In addition, holistic diagnostic techniques have been evaluated and are generally worthless. To name the most common examples, muscle testing (in which patients' arm muscles supposedly weaken from contact with an allergenic food) and cytotoxic screening (in which allergenic foods cause patients' blood cells to explode) are no more accurate than rolling dice. The conventional critique stops here, having once again made an entire class of patients the purview of the psychiatrist.

What has been ignored are the thousands of personal testimonials by people who have slowed or even arrested various degenerative conditions by altering their diet to avoid certain foods. It is likely that the glib explanations offered by holistic practitioners are worthless. It is equally likely that the equally glib dismissals by regular doctors of this body of evidence are premature. It is certainly possible that all these stories are yet another example of the power of the placebo effect, but this has not yet been proven. It is just as possible that there is a class of interactions between food and disease that are not yet acknowledged or understood by science.

The lesson for those of us who are struggling to find ways to heal is that experimenting with our diets may be useful but that *anyone's* explanations should be taken with a grain of salt. The science of nutrition is not yet sufficiently advanced for anyone to authoritatively state what a change in diet will or will not do for any given individual. The difficulty of making authoritative statements about nutritional matters is compounded by the extreme differences which are possible between people. Roger Williams, a researcher who discovered one of the vitamins of the B-complex, called this the principle of biochemical individuality. He proved several decades ago that the requirements for any given nutrient might vary by a factor of five or even ten times between members of the same species (Williams 50).

We should, therefore, give up on the goal of achieving someone else's idea of an "optimum" diet, whether that someone be Dean Ornish or a U.S. Senate Subcommittee. Instead, we should assess our own unique needs and vulnerabilities and be willing to experiment until we find a diet which helps us feel good and stay healthy. We can survey both conventional and alternative thinkers for ideas, and we should pay close attention to the available epidemiological evidence, but we should always remain aware that a particular recommendation may or may not apply to us.

The closest thing to a universal rule, supported by essentially all of the available evidence and agreed to by almost everyone, is the recommendation to eat more fruits and vegetables. By increasing fruits and vegetables in the diet one can increase the intake of vitamins, minerals, and fiber, and by displacing other less nutritious foods, lower the intake of fat and sugar. In addition, researchers are becoming increasingly interested in certain non-nutrient compounds in plants, called phytochemicals, which appear to offer health benefits even though they are not required in the diet. Whatever the reason, the epidemiology is clear. The more fruits and vegetables you eat, the lower your chance of contracting heart disease or cancer.

Even here, though, individual sensitivities are possible. Some people with severe carbohydrate intolerance may have trouble with the sugars in fruits. This may be why some people with depression report that their symptoms are exacerbated by bananas, a very high sugar fruit.

Similarly, some arthritis patients believe that their condition is worsened when they eat the so-called "nightshade" vegetables like tomatoes and potatoes. Though the actual incidence of these kinds of sensitivities is unclear, one should always remain aware of the possibility.

If we are willing to accept a somewhat lower level of proof than that offered by the case for fruits and vegetables, there are other reasonably conservative changes we can try. The most common conventional advice is to lower the fat content of the diet. While it seems unlikely that this would lengthen life significantly for most of us, it is still a very good idea for anyone suffering from or at risk for any of the diseases linked to dietary fat. This includes heart disease and some cancers (though probably not breast cancer). Some investigators would include diabetes on this list, though the evidence seems even weaker here.

Those scientists who are building a case for carbohydrate sensitivity or Syndrome X have begun to identify certain clues that someone may suffer from this condition. If an individual combines high blood pressure, high triglycerides, and a large waist when compared to hip size (i.e. a pot belly), then they may have trouble with sugars (Reaven 948-952). Skin tags on the neck and in the armpits have also been linked with a disordered sugar metabolism (Agarwal and Nigam 132-133). Anyone with these signs may wish to experiment with limiting sugar and possibly other refined carbohydrates like white flour.

Other recommendations which should probably be ranked at a lower tier of probability would include lowering salt, increasing fiber, and lowering caffeine. Interestingly, almost all of these recommendations can be accomplished by following what might be termed a traditional health food diet. This has been the most common approach to diet in alternative circles for many decades. This diet is nominally, but usually not perfectly, vegetarian. It emphasizes avoiding processed foods and seeking out foods that are as close as possible to the state of nature, such as whole grains or organic produce. Frequently supplemental foods like wheat germ or brewer's yeast are added to the diet. This kind of diet allows one to avoid micromanaging the various constituents of food. Instead of counting fat grams or calories or exchanges, one simply seeks out as many high quality unrefined plant foods as one can work into one's diet.

The only cautionary note necessary with this approach is to practice moderation. It is likely that severely restrictive diets are detrimental in wasting diseases like cancer and AIDS, and they may not be good for anyone. Many people involved in alternative cancer therapies were shocked and upset when The New England Journal of Medicine published a study in 1991 which evaluated the survival of cancer patients attending the Livingston-Wheeler Clinic, a well known alternative treatment center (Cassileth 1180-1185). Though patients at the Livingston Clinic had a survival rate roughly equivalent to those receiving conventional treatment, their quality of life was lower than the conventionally treated patients.

Given that conventional cancer therapies are not known for increasing quality of life, these results were disturbing to many people sympathetic to alternative approaches. It had become a cliche to refer to regular oncology as slash and burn medicine, and many observers assumed that alternatives were at least gentler and easier on patients, even if their effectiveness had not been demonstrated. Why, then, did quality of life scores indicate that conventionally treated patients were more comfortable?

The most likely explanation is that the restrictive vegetarian diet required by almost all alternative approaches to cancer was not only unsatisfying and hard to follow but did not provide enough calories to slow the wasting which is a hallmark of cancer. Cancer patients almost certainly benefit from a diet which has more vegetables and less fat than the average American diet, but some stringent vegan diets intended for "detoxification" are simply too rigorous for people battling a life threatening disease. It seems likely that AIDS patients on these diets would suffer in the same way as the Livingston cancer patients. No one with a wasting disease should lower their calorie intake to comply with anyone's miracle diet. Instead, the object should be to keep calorie intake up for as long as possible.

In fact, it is becoming increasingly clear that restrictive diets are counterproductive for almost everyone. In the Livingston Clinic diet, the decrease in calories was an accidental byproduct of the limited number of foods allowed on the diet, but many of us limit our calories deliberately. This is a bad idea, for both physiological and psychological reasons. Physiologically, the body responds to a severe decrease in calories by slowing metabolism to preserve tissue from the "famine" (Bennet and Gurin 84-85). Metabolic efficiency increases dramatically so that the body can burn as few calories as possible until food supplies are restored. Unfortunately, these adaptations continue after the diet ends. After dieting, the body needs fewer calories to sustain itself, so the unhappy dieter will be forced to limit food forever to maintain any weight loss.

Psychologically, those of us who struggle with our weight know what happens when we attempt to severely limit the quantity of food we allow ourselves, or when we decide that a favorite food is now bad and forbidden. Our resolve is inevitably followed by a counter-reaction, when we end up indulging ourselves more than if we had left well enough alone. In a way, the number one cause of binging is dieting. It is far healthier to make gradual incremental changes in our diet and indulge ourselves occasionally so that we don't feel deprived. This way we don't build up so much resentment, frustration, and hunger that the end of our diet is only a matter of time.

No matter what kind of diet we adopt, we cannot achieve perfect health through diet alone. Diet modification does not normally cure serious disease without other therapeutic interventions. Claims of miracle cures through magic diets should be taken with a grain of salt.

At the same time, a good diet is unquestionably the foundation of health. Whatever other therapies we receive, a good diet will strengthen us so that we can respond and heal vigorously. If we wish to get or stay well, a good diet is not optional.

6

ORTHOMOLECULAR NUTRITION

It is likely that in one hundred years it will seem odd that vitamin and mineral supplementation was ever ranked among the alternatives. This does not mean that the medical science of the future will have accepted all of the supplementation practices currently used in alternative circles. Many of these practices are almost certainly ineffective. Even the useful supplements will need to shake their association with overblown claims of effectiveness before they can take their place within the conventional therapeutic armamentarium.

Instead, it means that the distinction between supplements and conventional science is a somewhat artificial one. Alternatives like traditional Chinese medicine or homeopathy are truly alternative. They provide an overarching framework for understanding health and illness that does not rely on the foundational assumptions of Western science. In their pure, classical forms they require that a choice be made between their approach and conventional medicine at the outset. Attempts to graft them on to conventional medicine as "complementary" therapies are somewhat strained as long as their original vision remains intact.

In contrast, supplements are a product of Western science. It was Western science at its most reductionist which broke food apart into its various constituents and identified those essential to the health of human beings. It was Western science which learned to synthesize the essential compounds so that they could be manufactured and sold in supplemental form. Vitamin pills are as much a product of science as are penicillin or bypass surgery.

There are a variety of reasons why the sophisticated technology of nutrient supplementation ended up in the alternative ghetto. Conventional medicine is oriented towards the discovery of "magic bullets" against disease. The highest ideal of conventional medical research is to understand a problem so thoroughly that a drug can be inserted into precisely the right point in the human biochemistry to arrest the disease process. Doctors want drugs that are precisely targeted and highly effective. The more dramatic an effect they produce the better.

The only condition for which nutrients are magic bullets are the deficiency diseases like scurvy, beri-beri, or pellagra. Doctors satisfied themselves that this was the case in the first half of the twentieth century as the vitamins were discovered. Physicians reasoned that if a given disease didn't result directly from the lack of a vitamin at its proper spot in the body's web of biochemical reactions, then a vitamin or other nutrient could have no therapeutic effect. This became the mainstream consensus, and for many decades physicians repeated with near unanimity that vitamins were only useful in cases of clear deficiency.

This left mavericks and lay people who didn't know better as the only experimenters willing to tinker with vitamins. Over the years they began to report benefits from supplements in a variety of conditions. In a process which should now be familiar, conventional doctors attributed this to the placebo effect and focused their efforts on demonstrating that vitamin advocates simply didn't understand biochemistry very well. In many, though not all cases this was true, but of course it did not speak to the validity of their observations.

In the 1960s and 70s, the vitamin issue became tied up with larger issues of medical authority and the cultural significance of medicine. Two distinctly different models of how medicine should be practiced competed for the allegiance of the public. The older model was a product of the medical establishment. In it, the role of the physician is to identify the precise physiological abnormality or malfunction afflicting a patient and correct it with drugs or surgery. The patient's symptoms may provide clues, but the real key to success is the physician's skill at assembling the findings of the physical exam and any tests which have been ordered into a picture of the disease. The patient's experience of the disease is secondary.

This model has several consequences. Since the physician's role is to identify and treat disease, prevention of disease is almost always a secondary concern. Physicians focus on people who are already sick, and given the almost infinite number of ways the human frame can go wrong, the diagnosis and treatment of disease is as difficult and technical a discipline as human beings have developed. This forces the patient into a passive role. He or she provides the problem which the physician solves, but as a lay person the patient lacks the technical knowledge to contribute to the problem's solution. The solutions themselves are highly specific. Good drugs treat specific diseases by making exactly the right change to affect that disease. There is no room in this model for tonics or drugs that increase nonspecific resistance.

As a result of the social upheaval of the 60s and 70s, a new model began to compete with this one. In keeping with the general rejection of authority common during these decades, medical authority was rejected as well. People were now going to be responsible for their own health. Prevention was primary, through diet, exercise, stress control, and alternative therapies. The doctor would serve chiefly as a teacher, showing patients how to keep themselves healthy. Since it was assumed that individuals were generally good and institutions were generally evil, there was much interest in social causes of disease like bad air, bad water, or bad food.

Both of these models have something useful to offer. Neither one can replace the other. We need whole grains and CAT scans, health clubs and hospitals. The unfortunate antagonism between the two camps has done neither one any good. The hostility has kept potentially invaluable therapies, like vitamins and other supplemental nutrients, from being properly examined for at least two decades two long. Both sides share responsibility for this debacle.

The medical establishment once again suffered from a bad case of the "not invented here" syndrome, and showed its usual resistance to therapies which increase a person's ability to resist disease rather than attacking a disease directly. The alternative community just as characteristically touted supplements as panaceas before there was sufficient evidence to justify that kind of claim. Vitamins were a part of food, corporations had stripped from our diet in the name of profit, and doctors didn't like them. That was all the proof that seemed necessary.

Worst of all, both sides allowed the issue to be framed in terms of a dichotomy between vitamins and drugs, or even more broadly construed, between prevention and treatment, as if the use of one would automatically exclude the other. Doctors reacted with anger to the idea that anything purchased in a health food store could be as useful as their beloved pharmaceuticals. Members of the alternative community frequently acted as though any trip to an M.D. was an act of treason. Both sides were occasionally known to refuse treatment to a suffering patient unless he or she recanted any allegiance to the other side.

The standoff only began to break down when a plausible explanation for the success of nutrient therapy began to emerge. As discussed in chapter one, the scientific community generally will not accept anecdotes and testimony as evidence unless they seem plausible, and plausibility requires that a phenomenon make sense in light of what is already known. In practice this means that an effect must have at least a theoretical mechanism of action before it will be taken seriously. The free radical theory of Denham Harman provided that mechanism of action for megavitamin therapy.

Harman, a medical researcher at the University of Nebraska, was originally interested in the problem of aging, though his theory was later extended to a variety of other conditions as well. It was well known that normal metabolism tended to produce energetic, highly reactive molecular fragments as a byproduct. These fragments, known as free radicals, were not known to have any particular significance though it was clear that they were unavoidable. Harman, noting that free radicals engaged in uncontrolled and potentially damaging reactions with whatever molecules they in contact, began to wonder if free radicals might not cause gradual cumulative damage to the body's structures over time. Through a series of experiments beginning in the nineteen sixties, he demonstrated, at least to his own satisfaction, that free radicals were responsible for aging and many of the degenerative diseases associated with aging.

Over the next few decades, Harman's theory gradually won more and more adherents. Other researchers began to sketch in the details, showing how free radical reactions might play a role in many different diseases. As an example, it was shown that cholesterol was far more damaging to arteries when it had been altered, or oxidized, by free radicals.

These dangerous reactions could be controlled by a class of chemicals known as antioxidants. In one of the little ironies of history, Harmon had begun his experiments by extending the life of lab animals with common food preservatives like BHA and BHT. As experimenters moved closer to human trials with antioxidants, they de-emphasized these synthetic chemicals in favor of natural compounds whose toxicities were thought to be better understood. These natural antioxidants included vitamin C, vitamin E, the mineral selenium, and the provitamin beta carotene.

Suddenly the idea of taking vitamins in quantities much larger than one could conceivably consume in the diet didn't seem quite so wacky. Evidence began to accumulate that high doses of some vitamins might have profoundly beneficial effects in some conditions. A growing number of physicians began to suggest vitamins to their patients when the evidence for a specific application seemed particularly strong, for instance, the use of vitamin E in cardiovascular disease. An equally large number insisted on waiting until conclusive evidence from double-blind controlled trials was available.

This is where things stand today. Supplements appear to be moving toward acceptance by the conventional medical community, but several hurdles remain. There are large blinded trials in progress to test several antioxidant nutrients, but until the results of these trials are released, we must make educated guesses on the basis of the evidence we already possess. Even when the trials are complete, they have generally been designed to test one or two nutrients at one dose in a group of patients that share common characteristics. We can expect years of debate about the applicability of their findings to other combinations of nutrients at other doses in other types of people.

When all is said and done, it seems most likely that at least some vitamin therapies will prove to have value. There is so much evidence pointing in this direction that any other conclusion will not just be a surprise, it will produce a major shakeup in the emerging understanding of degenerative diseases as free radical processes. The conventional medicine of the future will almost certainly make use of a wide variety of supplemental nutrients.

The problem is that we don't know exactly which nutrients they will be. We can expect some surprises as the various possibilities are tested. This has already been made obvious by the results of the first large trials to be completed.

These trials tested the effects of beta carotene, a plant pigment which the body can convert into vitamin A. Beta carotene had long been viewed by mainstream scientists as one of the most promising candidates for the chemoprevention of cancer and heart disease. A truly enormous body of epidemiological evidence linked the consumption of large amounts of carotene rich vegetables to lower rates of disease.

It was thus a shock to the scientific community when three separate trials, released within a few months of each other, showed no beneficial results whatsoever from beta carotene supplements (Omenn et al. 1150-1155; Hennekens et al. 1145-1149; Alpha Tocopherol, Beta Carotene Cancer Prevention Study Group 1029-35). There were even hints that beta carotene might be dangerous to smokers. Beta carotene was a bust.

Members of the alternative community reacted with near hysteria to these findings. They produced a flurry of articles and news releases defending beta carotene. There were a variety of arguments—the trials weren't long enough, the experimental subjects weren't healthy enough to benefit (?), the beta carotene was synthetic rather than natural and might have been contaminated. There were even dark hints that the whole thing was part of a conspiracy by the pharmaceutical industry to destroy vitamin supplements as a potential rival. No one seemed willing to consider the obvious possibility that beta carotene simply wasn't the protective component in vegetables.

The news media reacted with headlines like "Are Vitamins Still Worth Taking?" and stories that called into question the whole process of scientific investigation, at least when health advice was involved. Reporters leaped to the conclusion that since beta carotene had failed, the active ingredient or ingredients in vegetables would never be isolated and that one could only improve one's health by eating real vegetables. The story became a morality play in which supplement users were portrayed as having been tempted by laziness into an attempt to circumvent the laws of good health and righteous living. Now they had received their comeuppance, while good folk who had persevered with plain food and vigorous exercise would go on to a sturdy old age.

This was an interesting example of role reversal. By emphasizing the magical qualities of living food, qualities which would always disappear if an attempt was made to extract them chemically, the news media was taking a vitalist position. It was supplement advocates who implied that the protection provided by fruits and vegetables was purely chemical in nature and could in principle be isolated by the techniques of scientific analysis. If beta carotene didn't work, some other pill or combination of pills would.

Christians need not reject vitalist arguments out of hand, so the "magic vegetable" argument is at least worth considering. It is at least possible that whole foods have effects other than chemical effects. At the same time, human beings have an enormous amount of practical experience with chemical and mechanical manipulations of foodstuffs which do change the health effects of foods. Cooking, milling, and fermenting all change the effect of food on the body, and none of these require a vitalist explanation. The isolation of vitamins and their effect on deficiency diseases demonstrates that in at least some cases powerful effects on the body can be traced to the presence or absence of a single chemical in food.

In the specific case of the chemoprotective effect of fruits and vegetables, one would have to ask why the protection afforded by these foods against different diseases seems to vary with the amounts of certain specific constituents of those foods if the effect is not chemical. Chemoprevention may be a very complicated process, involving many compounds in specific ratios, but there seems to be no reason to assume that the nature of the relationships won't eventually be untangled.

If the relationships are clear then we can make use of them. God has given us all foods, and that includes the constituents of those foods. There is certainly no theological reason to object to the isolation of a specific component of food to achieve a given end. There is no difference in principle between the use of a vitamin and the use of the bran produced by the milling of wheat to relieve constipation. Both involve the use of a dietary constituent in amounts larger than those typically consumed to achieve a therapeutic effect. Both are licit and useful.

Supplemental nutrients have some real advantages as therapeutic agents. Since they are compounds which are normally found in the body, in general they have less toxicity and produce fewer side effects than conventional drugs. This is the reason Linus Pauling termed nutritional therapies "orthomolecular", meaning "right molecule". Ideally, nutritional therapies do provide exactly the molecule the body needs, in contrast to "toximolecular" therapies which attempt to manipulate body processes by adding chemicals not normally found in human beings.

This argument does have its limits. Nutrients do have toxicities, and some nutrients can be dangerous in quantities only a few times larger than those commonly consumed in supplements. Vitamins A and D and the mineral iron are especially capable of causing problems. Despite this caveat, it remains true that nutrients are almost always easier on the body than pharmaceutical drugs. The body has biochemical machinery in place for handling a wide range of possible intake amounts of nutrients, and this may or may not be true of the creations of a pharmaceutical laboratory.

Nutrients are also generally cheaper than drugs. They are not subject to patent protection, so there is competition among numerous manufacturers. This kind of competition almost always lowers prices.

Unfortunately, the lack of patent protection also deprives nutrition researchers of a major source of research funding. Much pharmaceutical research is driven by the desire to find compounds which are both useful and patentable, so that a company can recoup its investment in research through a monopoly on the resulting drug. No one wants to do research which might encourage physicians to prescribe a competitor's product.

Members of the alternative community sometimes make too much of this. Alternative writers frequently imply that little or no medical research is conducted without the approval of the pharmaceutical companies. This is simply not true. While there is such a thing as a "medical industrial complex" it is more a community united by common interests than a monolith under unified control. There are numerous sources of research funding which have no connection with the pharmaceutical companies. This is why large trials have been funded to test vitamins and drugs no longer under patent, such as aspirin. Pharmaceutical companies do have an impact on the direction medical research takes, but they do not control it. Vitamin research does progress, but it does so somewhat more slowly than research in more heavily funded areas.

This is a problem for those of us who are attempting to make decisions about nutritional therapies. We would obviously prefer to have the authoritative information provided by large double-blind trials, but this won't be available for several years. The advantages of nutrient therapies are compelling enough that we may not want to wait until the final word is in. We have to weigh the available evidence and make the best decision we can.

The decision we make will depend upon the level of risk and uncertainty we are willing to accept. This will vary from person to person. Indeed, it may well vary for the same person at different times, depending upon the circumstances they face. For instance, a healthy person may find the unknown but probably minimal hazard posed by ten grams of vitamin C a day more risk than he or she is willing to accept for an uncertain benefit. If, however, that same person is diagnosed with cancer or AIDS, then the balance shifts. The clear and deadly hazard posed by a disease for which there is no fully satisfactory conventional treatment is a more immediate threat than the potential hazards of supplements. Suddenly, taking ten grams of vitamin C a day seems like a very reasonable gamble.

It is not just our own assessment of risk that may vary between preventive and therapeutic applications of nutrients. Frequently the amount of available information differs as well. It is easier to measure a therapeutic effect in a group of people who already have a disease than it is to test a compound's ability to prevent a disease in a group of healthy people. To test prevention one must start with people who might or might not get sick even without the intervention, so the group of subjects must be very large to show a clear effect. This means big trials that run for many years and cost a lot to administer.

For this reason, the science concerning therapeutic applications of nutrients is more mature than that of prevention. It is also almost unknown among conventional physicians. There are a whole series of nutrients which have shown clear benefits for certain diseases in good solid trials, but they are almost never utilized by M.D.s. Among these are CoQ10 for congestive heart failure (Soja and Mortensen S159-S68), magnesium for migraine (Mauskop and Altura 24-27), vitamin E for patients with pre-existing heart disease (Stephens et al. 781-786, though negative studies also exist), B6 for PMS (Wyatt et al. 1375-1381), glucosamine and chondroitin for arthritis (McAlindon et al. 1469-75), and, yes, vitamin C for colds (Hemila 1-6).

All of these nutrients are worth using for the conditions listed, but with only one exception none of them is sufficiently potent to serve as the only therapy used for those conditions by most people. The one exception is the use of vitamin C for colds. Colds are mild and self-limiting without any treatment at all. Since conventional drugs provide symptomatic relief only, vitamin C is a very reasonable first-line therapy.

The other nutrient therapies listed serve best as an adjunct to conventional therapies. At a minimum, they may need to be combined with another nutrient or another alternative therapy, and even then conventional drugs should be available as backup. It remains true that the only diseases for which nutrients are magic bullets are deficiency diseases.

Most physicians, including those doing the research, regard therapies with this level of effectiveness as the next best thing to useless. Even when investigators produce a clear beneficial effect, they will often characterize their own results as disappointing, simply because nutrients do not produce the dramatic results of drugs. When the Harvard Heart Letter evaluated CoQ10 they put it this way: "As an analogy, think of coenzyme Q10 as a bicycle. It may help a person get from one place to another more quickly if that person has no other transportation. But if a person also has a car—in this case, effective conventional drugs—then the addition of the bicycle is not of any particular use." ("Coenzyme Q10: The Next Aspirin?" 6).

This, of course, misses the point. The car may be faster than the bicycle but it will never be as cheap. And, to stretch the metaphor a bit, the car will never provide as pleasant a ride. Physicians in general are not very sensitive to the importance of expense and side effects to patients. A low cost low risk treatment that may allow us to get by with lower doses of conventional medication is powerfully appealing to those of us who have to actually take the drugs doctors prescribe.

There are several good books available which can provide sound guidance about those nutrient therapies with significant scientific evidence for their effectiveness. In particular, the <u>Natural Health Bible</u> by Steven Bratman and David Kroll is noteworthy for its accuracy and its even-handed approach. Anyone being treated for a serious or troubling medical condition would do well to check this book to see if there is an orthomolecular therapy which might be of help.

Preventive applications of nutrients have received a great deal of attention over the last few years. These applications do present some unique problems. In therapeutic applications, our choice is often between a nutrient and a drug. The drug will almost always be significantly more toxic than the nutrient. With a preventive application, our choice is between taking a supplemental nutrient and taking nothing at all. Since we are talking about giving healthy people pills for the possibility of a benefit, many scientists have insisted that these applications meet the highest possible standard of evidence before we use them.

It is a difficult choice to make. We are weighing the unknown possibility of risk from a supplement against the potential harm of doing nothing to prevent a disease which may strike us later. The risk of harm from a supplement is almost certainly minimal but it is not zero, and unfortunately we don't yet know just how far above zero it is. We can calculate our chances of contracting some diseases, like heart disease, on the basis of established risk factors, but this is an assessment of probability only. Improbable events do occur. People with no risk factors do get sick, and people with every risk factor do sometimes stay healthy. In addition, our understanding of the risk factors for most diseases is not as advanced as it is for heart disease. There is no way we can know with certainty what the state of our health will be in the future.

We are struck weighing one unknown risk against another. Luckily there is enough evidence available that we can make an order of magnitude assessment of the relative degree of risk posed by our two possible courses of action. If we do supplement, then we are joining millions of people in the United States who have supplemented their diets with various vitamins and minerals for decades. Several epidemiological investigations have examined the health of supplement users versus nonusers (Enstrom 194-202; Stampfer et al. 1444-1449; Losonczy et al. 190-196). These studies have repeatedly shown that supplements are either beneficial or neutral in their effects. Though epidemiology can't definitively establish that a particular benefit is the result of a given factor, it is quite good at identifying hazards. As long as doses are reasonable, supplements are safe.

If, on the other hand, we choose not to supplement, we expose ourselves to an "average" risk of degenerative disease. All of us know someone who died prematurely from heart disease or cancer. This becomes increasingly common as we grow older. This is the hazard which is ignored by conservative analyses which argue that the use of supplements is premature until controlled trials have nailed down the exact level of benefit and risk. While we wait, some of us will get sick and some of us will die.

As the case for supplements becomes more compelling, some Christians have reservations. Interestingly, these reservations take two mutually exclusive forms. On the one hand, some Christians worry that the use of nutrients as therapeutic agents stems from an excessive regard for the "natural". They fear that this emphasis on nature hints at and may even lead to paganism.

While it is true that some health food store literature tends in this direction, the current case for supplements has nothing to do with nature worship. It stems directly from our growing understanding of the biochemistry of disease. The physicians and scientists who are conducting research on antioxidant vitamins and minerals are hard nosed and practical. They aren't interested in nutrients because they have a secret urge to hug a tree. They are interested in nutrients because nutrients are effective therapeutic agents. The modern use of nutrients has no more to do with paganism than hormone replacement therapy for menopause has to do with the worship of female fertility.

Other Christians worry that supplements aren't natural enough. They ask why God would have designed the human body so that it would benefit from doses of nutrients that couldn't possibly be obtained from food. Wouldn't He have made us so that our bodies would achieve maximum health with the foods He gave us?

In the same way we could ask why our bodies benefit from vaccinations, or antibiotics, or cholesterol lowering medication. None of these is available to us in the state of nature. Unfortunately, we are no longer in Eden. We live in a fallen world. There is no sin in using what we have to relieve suffering.

What then should we take? The simplest approach, and probably the closest one can get to zero risk from the supplements themselves, is to take one to two times the R.D.I. of those vitamins and minerals designated essential. This approach has shown a measurable effect on immune function in the elderly in a controlled trial (Chandra 1124-1127). Epidemiological evidence indicates that it will probably lower the incidence of cataract as well (Seddon et al. 788-792). At a lower level of probability, there is some evidence that the dose of B vitamins in a typical multi may lower heart disease somewhat by lowering the level of homocysteine (Homocysteine Lowering Trialists' Collaboration 894-898), a toxic metabolite in the blood.

On the downside, R.D.I. level supplementation does not have much of an antioxidant effect, so it will not provide the striking level of protection shown in some studies at higher doses. It also isn't quite as easy to do as one might think. Most formulas that attempt to cram a full day's intake into one tablet neglect calcium and magnesium, because these two minerals are required in larger quantities than the vitamins.

It is also common to scrimp on lesser known nutrients like biotin, chromium, or selenium. These three do have R.D.I. values assigned, so a high quality supplement should provide them.

It is very likely that one can add significantly to the protection afforded by this kind of formula by supplementing several of the anti-oxidant nutrients at higher doses. The nutrient that is closest to acceptance by physicians is vitamin E. There is a large, growing body of research which indicates, but does not yet prove, that E protects against cancer, heart disease, and many of the problems of aging. 100 I.U. is probably the threshold for a significant antioxidant effect, and many studies have used 400 I.U. Supplementation should not exceed 800 I.U.

Vitamin C is less accepted by the medical community but it is just as safe. Vitamin C has a bit of a P.R. problem among doctors. They still associate it with Linus Pauling and his occasionally overblown claims that C was a virtual panacea. This association has slowed the pace of research. Nonetheless there are many decades of experience with very large doses of C. Vitamin C is almost certainly safe and clearly beneficial in doses of up to 1 gram (1000 mgs.) a day, probably both safe and beneficial in doses up to 3 grams (3000 mgs.) a day, and likely safe though not as unambiguously beneficial in doses up to 10 grams (10,000 mgs.) a day. Over the years, the scientific community has raised a series of concerns about doses in these ranges, from kidney stones to the recent charge of a pro-oxidant effect. These concerns have been primarily theoretical, based on test tube chemistry rather than data on health outcomes from clinical trials. Epidemiology continues to show benefits from reasonably large doses (Enstrom 194-202), and there seems to be no compelling reason to doubt the safety of vitamin C.

This approach is not the final word in supplementation. As the science of orthomolecular nutrition advances, I will be very surprised if nutrients don't become generally accepted adjunct or supportive therapies for a variety of conditions. It also seems likely that state of the art preventive health care will move away from one-size-fits-all nutritional prescriptions. Instead, each person will receive an individual assessment of their biochemical weak points and recommendations for nutritional therapies to strengthen those points of vulnerability. This kind of tailored approach will not only prevent disease, it will do so in a way which will avoid drugs, surgery, and their attendant pain and side effects. Christians should not hesitate to take advantage of this technology as it becomes available.

7

HERBS

If there is any single therapy most commonly associated with alternative medicine, it is herbalism. Anyone who is known to be an advocate of alternative approaches will frequently be asked, "Say, you don't know of any herbs that might help with such and such, do you?" This will be asked even if the person being questioned is primarily an advocate of massage, or bodywork, or meditation, or some other non-herbal therapy. Herbs are regarded as the common denominator of the holistically inclined.

In many ways this is an accurate perception. Herbs are the closest thing to a universal medicine, not just for the alternative community but for most of the world's non-Western peoples even today. Even conventional Western medicine relies on plants more than most physicians would like to admit, though pharmaceutical companies generally process them into pills and capsules which conceal the fact that their contents might once have done something so unsophisticated as to actually grow in the ground.

This universality brings with it a corresponding diversity. Plants produce an astonishing variety of chemical compounds capable of affecting human physiology. Almost as varied are the human traditions describing how these plants should be used. There are almost as many different ways to practice herbalism as there are herbalists.

Though many people cherish a romantic image of a backwoods root doctor or wise woman, very few people in modern America obtain medicinal herbs from this kind of source. Herbs have become big business. It isn't even necessary to visit a health food store to obtain them.

Most of the large drug or discount store chains now carry at least a few of the more popular herbs, usually in capsule form.

These herbs can be a valuable resource for modern health care consumers, but only if they are used in the context of modern medical knowledge. One of the greatest barriers to the effective use of herbs is an overly romanticized, overly respectful attitude towards the herbal practices of our ancestors. This is a common failing of many current advocates of herbalism. The handbooks produced by some, though not all, of these advocates can be both scientifically and historically unreliable. These handbooks seem all too willing to mirror the popular image of historical herbalism as a gentle therapy curing disease with cups of fragrant soothing tea.

If we examine the folk herbalism of our own country in the nineteenth century and earlier we can see that this is a distorted image. Our ancestors battled a variety of potentially fatal illnesses which commonly produced frightening and dramatically debilitating symptoms. The usual medical instinct of mankind is to assume that powerful illnesses require powerful remedies, and our ancestors were no exception. They favored potent purgatives and emetics as medicines. Just because you were being treated by a wise woman didn't mean that the treatment would be easy or pleasant.

It is true that it was probably easier than that offered by the local regular doctor. Conventional physicians could and did add bleeding and salivating with toxic mercury compounds to the torments suffered by patients. Compared to this, a simple vomit and sweat might seem almost idyllic. Modern people, however, are somewhat more accustomed to comfort. If we were exposed to the all-out rigors of Thomsonian herbalism, for instance, we would probably feel as if we had been turned over to a Satanic tormenter.

Thomsonian medicine was a nineteenth century attempt to codify and regularize the herbal knowledge of American Indian healers. Samuel Thomson even provided a quasi-scientific explanation for the success of his therapy. He believed that all illness was the result of excessive cold in the body's interior, and that it could be dispelled by the application of sufficient heat. He therefore treated almost all ill-nesses with cayenne pepper, sweat baths, and the herb lobelia. The active ingredient in lobelia is chemically related to nicotine. It produces vomiting and profuse sweating. It is not gentle. Despite this, Thomso-nianism was enormously popular in the first half of the nineteenth cen-tury (Rothstein 45).

At least some of the popularity of Thomsonianism and other schools of herbal healing was probably earned. Most people before the twenti-eth century were loaded with parasites, and it is conceivable that a strong purgative might remove at least some of them. In addition, as previously proposed, sometimes any strong stimulus is enough to ini-tiate healing. If nothing else, the herbal therapies of our ancestors were certainly capable of providing a good swift kick to the body's systems. Unfortunately, most of us today aren't really interested in a good swift kick.

The popular understanding of the herbal traditions of other cultures is similarly misleading. The herbal pharmacopeias of China and India have been thoroughly mined for salable products by the health food industry, but as they are sold today they rarely lend themselves to their traditional applications. Both Traditional Chinese Medicine (usually abbreviated TCM) and the Ayurvedic medicine of India provide pre-scriptions that are highly individualized. Patients are analyzed in terms of basic natural forces as understood by Oriental philosophy and cos-mology. These forces have little or no relationship to Western con-cepts. Popular writers sometimes describe this as an analysis of "energy flow" in the body, but even this is a Western metaphor that doesn't really capture the Eastern understanding.

Once the practitioner has "diagnosed" the patient, he prescribes a complex mixture of herbs and other substances designed to influence this pattern in the direction of balance and health. This mixture may contain dozens of different herbs, and it will be unique to a particular patient. It is usually taken as a very strong tea. Since these teas are not compounded with taste in mind, they often have a pronounced medicinal flavor.

In contrast, Chinese herbs in the United States and Europe are generally mass-marketed as single herbs or as standardized formulas. Though there are some Chinese patent medicine formulas available, these are most popular among ethnic Chinese. Most of the Chinese herbs for sale in health food stores are produced by Western manufacturers for a Western market. As a result, the indications for use provided in promotional literature or (sometimes) on the bottles themselves are for symptoms and conditions that Western consumers find familiar. The concepts of Chinese medicine are either not present at all or they are seriously oversimplified.

The form in which the herb is administered is also different from the usual traditional forms. The Western market is split between teas that are as much beverages as medicines and dried powdered herbs in capsules. Western consumers raised on fruit juice and soda pop won't sit still for the bitter medicinal brews used by the Chinese. Western people expect medicine to come as pills or capsules, and manufacturers are happy to oblige.

In short, the herbalism readily available today cannot be precisely identified with any traditional system. It isn't the same as that practiced early in the history of the United States with both American and European plants. It isn't the same as any of the traditional medical systems of the East. It uses plants from all these traditions but it provides them in new forms and it adapts them, both to new applications and to a new, modern sensibility. As a result, we cannot rely on traditional practices to guide us, nor can we judge the new herbalism by the successes or failures of the old.

People turn to herbs today because they are looking for mild medicines with minimal side effects. They want a safe, cheap alternative for the self-care of minor illness. Traditional systems can't provide this, because they evolved with a different agenda. A new herbalism is evolving, however, which can.

At its best, the new herbalism draws on conventional medical and chemical knowledge as well as traditional indications. The marketplace has moved away from jars and bins of musty bulk herbs to standardized preparations packaged with the same care as conventional pharmaceuticals. Not only can one trust the larger companies to provide the plant they say they are providing, to an increasing degree one can find products with a standardized potency of the plant's active ingredients. This kind of preparation is as trustworthy as an aspirin, and frequently safer.

This change, not yet fully completed, has gone almost unnoticed. Critics of herbal medicine continue to attack herbs as inherently unreliable and unpredictable compared to the products of a pharmaceutical company, without noticing that the techniques pioneered by the pharmaceutical giants are now being applied to herbs. These same critics will accuse the herbally inclined of being simple-minded, since they equate "natural" with "safe". "Hemlock is natural," the critics hoot, "and look what it did for Socrates!" While this argument is a useful reminder that one should not stuff random plants into one's mouth while walking in the woods, it has no real relevance to commonly available medicinal herbs. The changes in the herbal marketplace have tended to remove the most toxic plants from ready availability. It is now necessary to really go looking to find a seriously dangerous plant.

It is true, though, that people are frequently drawn to herbs because of a preference for the natural. Just as is true in the case in dietary supplements, some Christians are suspicious of an undue fondness for the natural, since they associate this attitude with a creeping New Age paganism. The "naturalness" of herbs can actually keep these Christians away from them.

It should be clear that the herbs themselves are unquestionably licit. It has only been within the last century or two that anything other than herbs as medicines has been available to anyone anywhere. Medieval monasteries had herb gardens for medicinal purposes, not because the monks were gourmet cooks (though this, too, may have been true in some cases). As we read in Sirach 38.4, "The Lord created medicines out of the earth, and the sensible will not despise them." This includes those of us today.

The use of medicinal herbs is consistent with almost any set of beliefs. They were used by our ancestors because they produced a physiological effect on the body. At various times and places, plants have also been used as religious, mythological, or magical symbols, as has almost everything else in the natural world at one time or another. If a given plant has been used in this way, it does not mean that we are forbidden to take advantage of the physiological effect it produces. If we were, then the use of numbers in numerology would mean that we could no longer do arithmetic.

Herbs are useful today whether we are fond of the natural world or not. Modern standardized potency herbs fill some conspicuous gaps in the pharmacopoeia of conventional medicine, and any of us may find ourselves in need of something that can fill one of those gaps. The gaps exist because of the characteristics of modern medicine which have been discussed in the preceding chapters. Medicine as practiced today emphasizes therapies with dramatic effects and specific actions against particular pathogens or disease processes.

As a result, conventional medicine cannot provide much in the way of mild medicines. Even over-the-counter drugs are noteworthy for the number and variety of side effects they cause. While it would be foolish to assert that all herbs are free of side effects, there are commonly available herbs which can treat minor health problems while providing fewer side effects than the conventional drugs usually used for those problems.

The best example is the use of echinacea for colds and flu. Echinacea is so good that many people have a hard time believing it even after they have tried it. It combats minor viral conditions by producing a potent nonspecific stimulation of the immune system (Weiss 229-230). In contrast to over-the-counter cold medicines, which produce comfort only without affecting the course of the illness, echinacea actually improves the body's ability to fight the virus. Anyone who honestly experiments with tincture of echinacea will quickly realize that while it may not cure a cold in the way antibiotics cure a bacterial infection, echinacea can dramatically shorten the length of time one suffers. And it does this without any noticeable side effects whatsoever.

Echinacea is also a good example of the way herbs can fill a second prominent gap in the conventional armamentarium. Conventional medicine is good at destroying pathogens, but bad at strengthening particular body functions. In the case of a disease like the common cold, in which medicine is powerless to destroy the invading organism, physicians are reduced to manipulating symptoms. In contrast, herbalism offers a huge variety of tonics, or in Oriental terms, "harmony remedies" capable of improving the body's response to various stressors.

Not all of these herbs have been examined as carefully by scientists as we might wish. This isn't necessarily because they don't work, but because this kind of drug activity has not been regarded as useful or interesting by researchers until very recently. This is not pure prejudice, since the historical record clearly shows that the herbal approach is not as successful in dealing with life threatening illness as is the more focused approach of conventional medicine. There are attacks on the body which the body simply isn't capable of overcoming on its own, no matter how many supplements and herbs we consume. When we face this kind of attack, we can be glad that scientific research has focused on ways to destroy the attacker.

Still, we frequently face illnesses which don't fall into this kind of life or death category. When we have a minor virus, or a minor disruption in our body's smooth functioning caused by simple wear and tear, the herbal approach allows us to tweak our body's responses a bit. Once one has become accustomed to using a few simple, reliable herbs in this way, minor health problems which would previously have required a physician can be handled at home.

There are a number of herbs which have been investigated thoroughly enough to ensure both safety and effectiveness. Ginger, in capsules, tea, or candied form, is a remarkably effective treatment for nausea and migraine headache (Bone et al. 669-671). Garlic, in at least some forms, has a protective effect on blood vessels, though this is probably not because of an effect on serum cholesterol (Efendy et al. 37-42; Koscielny et al. 237-49). Saw palmetto extract can relieve a swollen prostate as effectively as the prescription drugs usually used for this purpose (Plosker and Brogden 379-395). An extract of milk thistle seeds can strengthen liver function enough to enable this organ to withstand a variety of insults (Flora et al. 139-143). Valerian is a safe sedative and sleep aid (Lindahl and Lindwall 1065-1066).

Some knowledge is necessary to use these herbs safely and effectively, as is true for any medicinal substance. The most common error is to use herbs as a dietary supplement on an ongoing basis rather than as a medicine for a specific time-limited condition. This is one of the few disadvantages of the modern herb marketplace. Though herbs in capsules are easier to take than the teas or tinctures our ancestors relied upon, this very ease of use can encourage a thoughtless or irresponsible approach. It is all too easy to include a few herb capsules in one's daily handful of vitamin supplements with the assumption that they function in basically the same way.

This can lead to low level liver toxicity over the long run. Our ancestors were less likely to experience this kind of complication, both because of the difficulty of preparing and consuming the herbs they used and because of the seasonal availability of most medicinal plants. These limitations have been erased by the easy year-round availability of encapsulated herbs. Some herbs are particularly toxic to the liver, and are best completely avoided. These include comfrey (when used internally), coltsfoot, germander, and possibly chapparal. Other herbs should be used to treat specific problems and then discontinued when the problem resolves. The only herbs which can be safely used on an ongoing basis are herbs with a history of use as foods in addition to their use as medicines. These plants, such as garlic or bilberry (European blueberry), are safe to use every day.

Even with purely medicinal, non-food plants, it is best to limit oneself to herbs with a long history of human use. These are the plants whose strengths, weaknesses, and dangers are likely to be reasonably well understood, even if they have not been examined by biomedical science with the detail we might like. We can be fairly confident of our knowledge of their medicinal virtues, simply on the basis of centuries of empirical evidence. Unfortunately, there are no miracle cures among them.

There is something about herbs that triggers wild enthusiasm for their ability to cure the incurable. It seems at least plausible that some previously unknown plant might hold the key to a killer disease. If we are told that disease can be cured by colored light, or that our bowels are packed full of years' worth of feces, most of us are understandably skeptical; but if we are told that some tropical explorer has found a cure for cancer in the remote jungle, this seems almost reasonable.

Herb marketers are more than willing to take advantage of this kind of hope. As a result, every few years a new miracle plant is touted. These frequently come from tropical areas, which increases their allure given our fascination with the exotic mysteries of the rainforest. For a few months at least, anecdotal reports will tell of miraculous cures resulting from the use of the plant. These stories will usually center on cancer.

The perennial appeal of herbal cancer cures stems from an unpleasant fact, which no one wants to face squarely. There is as yet no good answer to cancer. Conventional treatment is painful and debilitating and not very effective. Alternative treatment may or may not be painful and debilitating, but it isn't very effective either. Everyone wants to find a simple treatment which is easy to use and miraculously effective, but the best available evidence indicates that it doesn't exist. Given the complexity of the problem of cancer, it may never exist.

This doesn't mean herbs are useless in the face of serious disease, but it does mean that they should be limited to use as supportive adjunct therapies. In the case of cancer, there are several herbs which can be used to maintain immune function during chemotherapy. The best of these is probably astragalus (Wang 180-183), though some Western authorities argue that the largely Chinese research on this plant needs to be confirmed before it can be fully accepted. There may also be a role for one or more of the fungal drugs from the Oriental traditions, such as reishi or maitake (Wang et al. 699-705), though the same caveat applies here as well.

Beyond this, the cancer patient tempted by an exotic herb should again remember that he or she is weighing unknown risk against potential benefit. This must always be an individual decision, but it may be useful to note that both risk and benefit are particularly uncertain in the case of a tropical plant. Many of the therapies used by alternative healers, such as nutrient supplements, have enough of a history of epidemiological investigation that we can at least make an order of magnitude assessment of hazard. This is not true for medicinal plants which are new to the Western market. Even traditional use by indigenous people isn't a perfect guide, since one can never know how accurately the tradition has been transmitted to the Western consumer. In general, one should always experiment cautiously, remaining sensitive to the reactions of one's own body.

In contrast to modern oncology, modern cardiology is quite good. Though there are herbs which may have a mild beneficial effect in heart disease, none of them can equal the power of conventional treatment. Heart patients who wish to experiment with herbs could reasonably consider hawthorne, garlic, and ginger for their positive influence on blood pressure, cholesterol, and blood clotting, but in no case should they be substituted for a prescribed conventional medication. The decline in heart disease deaths over the last few decades is largely due to modern medicine (Hunink et al. 535-542), and it would be foolish to deprive oneself of the benefits available through modern treatment.

The only other killer disease for which herbs should be considered as a primary treatment is senility, either Alzheimer's Disease or cerebrovascular arteriosclerosis. Though there is no herbal treatment which can cure or arrest these diseases, a standardized potency extract of gingko biloba leaves can slow their progression (Le Bars et al. 1327-1332). The effect is not dramatic, but it is present, and gingko has essentially no toxicity. It can cause headaches in a few susceptible people, but it is otherwise completely safe to experiment with. Since there is no danger involved, the relatively modest benefit which gingko can provide may be worth pursuing.

Most of us don't need miracles. Almost all of us, however, can find a use for time-tested low-tech medicines that can safely relieve the irritating symptoms that all of us experience at one time or another. Standardized potency herbs from reliable suppliers can meet this need in a way that has no real equivalent in conventional medicine. Herbs are a blessing from God, and we should use them gratefully.

8

TRADITIONAL CHINESE MEDICINE AND AYURVEDA

For those Americans who were not directly involved in the counterculture during the nineteen sixties, the more exotic forms of alternative medicine were largely invisible. Such traditions as homeopathy and chiropractic were still present, but they were generally viewed as dying if not already dead. The long history of these systems in America was in some ways a barrier to their acceptance, since they were viewed as remnants of a pre-scientific age. It was not until the public was startled by the success of an exotic newcomer that other alternative systems could gain a hearing.

That "newcomer" was Traditional Chinese Medicine, often abbreviated TCM. When Nixon made his trip to China in the early nineteen seventies, his press contingent included James Reston of the New York Times. While in China, Reston was struck by appendicitis. After Chinese physicians performed an emergency appendectomy, Reston received several acupuncture treatments for pain. Reston was intrigued by the use of this ancient therapy in a modern hospital, and after his recovery he wrote a front page article about the experience for the Times (Reston 1). In this article he noted that, however it worked, the acupuncture had successfully relieved his pain.

Reston had provided the right catalyst at the right moment. Acupuncture changed from an obscure topic of study by scholars of ancient Chinese thought to a focal point of popular fascination. Suddenly, there were articles and news stories on acupuncture everywhere. Within a few years, there were Americans studying TCM in China, and not long after that there were training programs available in the United States. Acupuncture and other forms of TCM had become contenders in the American medical marketplace.

There are probably several reasons why TCM was so suddenly successful. The counterculture had already awakened an interest in Eastern thought. China had been a closed society for many years, and there was a natural curiosity about how it had developed. TCM itself had all the earmarks of an exotic secret discipline, almost occult in its reliance on slender needles, burning knots of mugwort and bizarre medicinal substances. Even better, this exotic magical science actually seemed to work, as declared by the ultimate organ of respectability, the New York Times. Perhaps most important of all, TCM didn't seem to require that Western scientific medicine be abandoned. Chinese hospitals appeared to have integrated the best of both traditions. Reston himself had received a conventional appendectomy before his acupuncture.

To a degree, this smooth integration of the two traditions was an illusion. Even in China, TCM and Western medicine operate in parallel more often than they work together (Eisenberg 156). This division is hard to avoid, as the two systems are built on entirely different conceptual frameworks. They are so different that real integration is very nearly impossible. It is possible to see the world as Western science sees it, or as the Chinese practitioners of TCM see it, but it is hard to see it both ways at the same time. This isn't necessarily because one is right and the other wrong, though that is one possible interpretation. The conflict arises at an earlier point, before truth or falsehood has even been addressed.

Chinese philosophers and Western scientists don't just disagree about what one sees when one looks at the world, they disagree about how one engages in the act of seeing. Where Westerners analyze and dissect, Chinese thinkers see wholes. Where Westerners see things, the Chinese see processes. Where Westerners draw divisions, the Chinese see continuity. Even something as self-evident to the West as the principle of non-contradiction is not assumed in the same way by the Chinese. It is a foundational assertion of Western thought that a proposition and its negation cannot be true at the same time. A and not-A cannot both be true. But to the Chinese, A contains not-A, and indeed is always in the process of becoming its own contrary.

This leads to an immediate problem for Christians, who can get thoroughly tied up attempting to decide if the Chinese philosophy at the heart of TCM is a denial of Christian truth, or if it is even answering the same questions. There are no clear or simple solutions to the dilemma. For instance, the Chinese analyze the ceaseless change and flow of reality in terms of yin and yang. Yin and yang are not absolutes but are instead qualities of relation. Things are yin or yang in relation to something else, so there is never yin without yang or yang without yin. Yin is dark, feminine, hidden, and yielding. Yang is light, masculine, emerging, and assertive. Both yin and yang contain the seed of their opposite and constantly flow into one another. The Chinese believe that this flow can be perceived in all things.

Is this religion, philosophy, or science? Is it all of the above or none of the above? Our answer may determine whether Christians can use Chinese medicine with a clear conscience. If Chinese medicine is built on the foundation of a non-Christian religion, then we would need to think long and hard before submitting to its ministrations.

At the most basic level, TCM as it is commonly found in the United States does not require that we honor or petition any foreign gods. We are not asked to participate in any specifically religious rituals. Though this is a somewhat minimal standard, it is still important to know that by these criteria TCM is not a religion.

Nor is it science as usually understood in the modern West. Though it is obviously based on detailed and sophisticated observation of man and nature, TCM lacks some crucial mechanisms that would allow this empirical knowledge to be assembled into a convincing description of nature's laws. China lacks a tradition of experimentation. In addition, there is no culturally acceptable way for TCM to remove false information from its storehouse of beliefs and techniques.

Both of these problems stem from the Chinese reverence for the wisdom of their predecessors. Maxine Hong Kingston's China Men contains a particularly revealing episode, when her mother scoffs at purported new knowledge by saying "Anything that necessary has to have been invented long ago" (Kingston 191). From the Chinese point of view, the older it is, the more authoritative it is.

We can only discover new knowledge if we are willing to test our assumptions and replace them when they are flawed. It is the great achievement of modern science to have institutionalized the process of experimentation and verification so that assumptions are tested and retested. This process is neither as neutral nor as effective as its apologists would have us believe, but it is certainly better than the reflexive deference to the opinions of the ancients which is characteristic of the Chinese.

Because of this deference, nothing is ever discarded in TCM. Over the centuries, TCM has become a huge unwieldy mishmash of startlingly effective therapies mixed with the useless or even dangerous. When the Chinese are wrong, they are sometimes very wrong. Some of TCM's traditional herbal prescriptions contain toxic heavy metals. Some of TCM's understanding of anatomy is simply not true, possibly because of the traditional prohibition against autopsy.

Most startling of all to the modern observer, all of TCM's myriad details are made to fit into an overall theoretical structure which is at least several millennia old. This structure is quite similar to others that arose at roughly the same time in other parts of the world. In common with TCM, the Ayurvedic medicine of India and the Hippocratic tradition of ancient Greece saw the world in terms of the movement and interaction of certain basic forces or elements. The Greeks, following Empedocles, proposed that the four primal constituents of reality were earth, air, fire, and water. The Chinese added metal to this list. These elements had their counterparts in the body, eventually named black bile, yellow bile, blood, and phlegm in the Greek tradition. In all of these traditions, health was conceived of as a state of balance between the body's different constituents or humors.

In its day, this was great science. In each of the cultures that developed some form of humoral medicine, this focus on natural forces replaced other, purely magical views. But, humoral medicine was abandoned by the West for a reason. As more and more was learned about the natural world, it became clear that the four elements and the four humors were insufficient to explain all the myriad phenomena that were being observed. Unfortunately, this process of experimentation and subsequent abandonment of discredited ideas is precisely the step the Chinese could not or would not take. They have been working with humoral medicine ever since.

The Chinese should receive credit for having constructed the most sophisticated variation on the basic humoral theme. The fluid, almost metaphorical elements that the Chinese saw underlying the world are unquestionably an improvement on the much more inert basic substances hypothesized by the Greeks. One reason TCM has lasted as long as it has is because it is a flexible and resilient system. Nonetheless, over the centuries the endless complications and details added to TCM have begun to resemble the desperate efforts of pre-Copernican astronomers to save an Earth-centered universe by adding additional planetary motions, or epicycles, to the perfect circular orbits imagined by Ptolemy. As the wheels within wheels multiply, one begins to wonder if perhaps the basic scheme shouldn't be rethought. What was once science has become something else, something which restricts progress rather than assisting it.

If, then, TCM is neither a religion nor a science, then what is it? It is best thought of as a central philosophical core encrusted over the centuries with the techniques discovered or developed by practicing physicians. The core itself is not in direct competition with Christianity, but Christianity can speak to some of the issues it raises.

For instance, TCM assumes that reality is ultimately one. If all things are in essence one, then distinctions are illusory. TCM works these implications out in careful detail, charting the processes by which one thing becomes another as their essential unity is revealed.

Christianity, however, reveals that some distinctions are not illusory—they are essential. The Creator will always transcend His creation. Within creation, God has delighted in distinctions, and some of them are intended for eternity. When history has reached its end, you and I will still be different people.

Other distinctions minimized by TCM also prove to be crucial. Light and dark are not equally real, as dark is the absence of light, not its counterpart or companion. Good and evil are not equivalent. The Chinese are not indifferent to evil, but Christian theology provides a more solid foundation for opposition to evil than does the philosophy of TCM.

But TCM is not wholly wrong. Just as Aristotle contributed to the development of Christian thought, the Chinese have much to offer to medicine. The diagnostic techniques that give Chinese physicians such a keen sense of the direction of change in living systems are worth examination. The emphasis on balanced functioning is a useful counterweight to the illness orientation of the West. And even some of the more controversial aspects of Chinese medicine, such as the vitalistic focus on the life force, or "chi", may be worth preserving.

Since chi is usually described as a form of life energy, it is often misunderstood in the West. It is this, but it is also much more. Those of us who think with the traditional categories of the West usually understand energy to be the opposite of matter. An energy unique to life sounds to us like some kind of spiritual force, since by definition, at least as we understand the definition, it cannot be a part of the material body. We can easily confuse the life force with the soul, and tampering with it starts to seem like occultism.

The Chinese conception may provide a way out of this dilemma. Once again, the Chinese don't draw the lines in the same place we do.

Chi is energy, yes, but this does not mean that it is completely immaterial. Chi is that which forms, shapes, and animates matter, and it can no more be present without matter than one side of a piece of paper can be present without the other. Chi is not limited to human beings, or even to living things. It is universal, present everywhere and in everything in a more or less refined form. When the Chinese describe it, at times chi seems as abstract as the ideal forms described by Plato. At other times it seems as mundane as if it were just a Chinese word for the calories we obtain from food or the oxygen we extract from the air.

Chi will probably never translate directly into a scientific term acceptable in the West, but much of what the Chinese conceptualize as chi has been neglected by the West, probably because we are sometimes too willing to draw sharp distinctions between such categories as matter and energy, or mind and body. Chief among these neglected aspects is a sense of form, of that which lends continuity despite ceaseless change. If, for instance, every molecule in our body is replaced over time, why are we recognizably the same person?

We don't necessarily need to postulate a life force to answer this question, but we will need to talk about pattern and configuration. To use a currently popular buzzword, we will need to talk about information. Living beings are enormously complex information processing systems. The information encoded in the genetic material imposes its own structure on the matter and energy the creature takes into itself, and these raw materials are transformed into a part of the creature's own life. The environment in which the creature lives is also packed with information, and a living being must constantly read these forms and patterns if it is to adapt to them and survive.

This endless flow of information is far more reminiscent of the flow of chi than of the more static model of the West. Though Western scientists should know better, they often seem to think of the body as a hairy bag of chemicals which can be manipulated with relative ease. The body, or better yet, the whole creature, is however endlessly adaptive and responsive. If we attempt to push it in a particular direction it will almost always push back.

It might be more fruitful to consider the possibility of a more subtle approach. Perhaps we could intervene directly in the information flow. Perhaps, rather than attempting to push bodily processes in a particular direction with brute force, we might simply send a message that the change is necessary, and allow the body to correct itself.

Here the Chinese are way ahead of us. All of the therapies of TCM are intended to balance the flow of chi and other basic forces through the body. Using herbs, massage, exercise, and acupuncture, the practitioner of TCM attempts to adjust the flow of the forces in the direction of harmony.

The complex herb mixtures which the Chinese use are probably best understood as drugs whose actions could in principle be explained by Western pharmacology. The mysticism and metaphor characteristic of Chinese thought don't seem to provide any compelling advantages in understanding the activity of herbs. Though these herbal mixtures may provide some real advantages in terms of mildness and lack of side effects, their mechanism of action is essentially the same as Western drugs.

Acupuncture, however, is another matter. Its mechanism of action, whether it is understood in Chinese or in Western terms, provides a unique drug-free way of intervening directly in the body's homeostatic mechanisms. The Chinese, of course, believe that the needles can fine-tune the flow of chi through the body's meridians, a system of pathways or channels whose existence is not accepted by most Western scientists. The scientific community prefers to explain acupuncture's activity as mediated purely by its effect on the nervous system. It has been demonstrated that the needles, whatever else they are doing, do cause the release of the body's natural pain relievers, the endorphins (Chao et al. H2127-34).

This has led to a focus on acupuncture anaesthesia among Western researchers. This function of acupuncture is the easiest to understand in Western terms, but it is not the most important use of the technique from the Chinese point of view. They use acupuncture to affect body functions in a variety of ways, not just to relieve pain.

Not all of these additional applications have been incontrovertibly demonstrated. Most of the research on these applications has been done by the Chinese themselves. Unfortunately, most Chinese research is still not up to Western standards. Whether it is from a lack of interest in jumping through hoops to satisfy the Western scientific community or from a simple lack of resources, the Chinese research agenda is more oriented towards practical applications than towards "proof".

As a result we really don't know what acupuncture's full range of utility is. It will be surprising, however, if the several millennia of practical experience accumulated by the Chinese prove to be the product of the placebo effect alone. It is possible, but it seems more likely that acupuncture will prove to have a wide range of effects on the human body.

This will provide a challenge to the Western scientific community. While the meridian system will probably never be scientifically acceptable, some means will need to be found to account for a range of dynamic, non-local effects that seem to be beyond the power of the endorphin hypothesis to explain. Acupuncture is inherently holistic because it relies on the body's own power to adjust and correct its own functioning in response to the proper message. Most conventional physicians aren't quite ready to trust the body this much yet.

This leaves those of us who are health care consumers in a familiar dilemma. We want the benefits of a non-drug therapy which may be able to stimulate healing in a way which is both safe and subtle, but there is no reliable information which can tell us how closely acupuncture approaches this ideal. We aren't comfortable abandoning our caution completely to put ourselves in the hands of a traditional practitioner. At the same time, we don't want to ignore a promising therapy of great potential power.

Luckily, TCM comes in a variety of forms. The completely traditional practitioner is not our only option. Though there is little interest in Chinese herbalism among conventional physicians, acupuncture is becoming increasingly respectable. As a result there are a growing number of "medical acupuncturists" trained in Western medicine but able to use acupuncture as a therapeutic option.

This emerging discipline isn't perfect. Since medical acupuncturists are generally committed to the endorphin model of acupuncture action, they tend to limit the applications of their therapy, focusing on pain and musculo-skeletal problems. Acupuncture is probably more powerful than this. But, a medical acupuncturist is unquestionably the safest way to take advantage of this therapy. He or she won't attempt to treat a condition with acupuncture which should be treated with conventional therapies, and he or she will avoid those Chinese therapies which might be hazardous.

Indeed, if at all possible one should receive acupuncture from a full-fledged M.D. or someone supervised by an M.D. This ideal is not always possible, but it is more possible with acupuncture than with most other alternative therapies. This is a good thing, since the huge mishmash of TCM contains techniques that are both more powerful and more dangerous than is typical in the alternative world.

Receiving acupuncture from someone whose background is in Western medicine also allows the Christian whose conscience is troubled by Chinese philosophy to avoid this problem altogether. Since Western physicians almost always assume that the Chinese explanation of their medicine is of little or no value, they tend to strip away any remnant of Chinese thought at the outset. Acupuncture becomes an empirically derived technique which can be exploited and investigated rather than a window into a world view.

There are other systems of traditional medicine becoming available in the United States which have not passed through this pruning process. The most prominent is Ayurveda, the medicine of India. Ayurveda is a much more recent arrival in the United States than is

TCM, but it has achieved a great deal of visibility very quickly. Much of this is because of the popularity of the writings of Deepak Chopra, a conventionally trained physician who returned to the medicine of his ancestors. His books combine the basic humoral framework of Ayurveda with a popularized version of Hindu religious thinking.

Chopra embodies the central difficulty of Ayurveda for Christians. Most Ayurveda is much more closely tied to the religious heritage of its homeland than is the case for traditional medical systems which have been in the United States longer. Indeed, most Ayurvedic practitioners have a direct connection with a single religious group, the Transcendental Meditation organization founded and led by Mahareshi Mahesh Yogi. Sooner or later most practitioners linked to this group will recommend TM to their patients.

This is not a form of cult recruitment. From the Ayurvedic perspective, attention to one's consciousness is a legitimate form of therapy. Since the TM organization is committed to the value of a particular form of meditation, it isn't surprising that its members rely on this method with their patients.

Unfortunately, the Christian understanding of the human spiritual condition differs from the Hindu. Hinduism, at least in the simplified form represented by TM, regards the problem of human unhappiness as one that stems from a lack of knowledge. Human beings fail to recognize their essential unity with God, who is immanent in the material world. This failure of perception can be remedied by training the consciousness until the true nature of reality is apparent. This process leads to peace.

In contrast, Christianity regards the break between God and human beings as far more radical in nature and as a result requiring a far more radical remedy. Sin has produced such a great gulf between human beings and God that no human action can enable us to cross it. We are lost unless God Himself provides us with a bridge to return to Him. That bridge is Jesus Christ. Only Jesus, both perfect man and the Divine Son, could accept the burden of our sin and restore our relationship with God. No matter how we meditate or train our consciousness, we cannot be free of that burden by our own efforts. Only God can save us.

Hinduism as filtered through TM is a religion of knowledge. We are saved by gaining the ability to know a truth which we did not know before. Christianity is a religion of grace. God, rather than the person, acts, and through God's act we are saved. Given this difference in goals, it would be surprising if the two faiths didn't offer different prescriptions.

The greatest fault of the TM organization is its tendency to present its prescription as a purely medical recommendation rather than a religious practice. TM has successfully sold its meditation system as nothing more than a way to achieve stress control and greater health. It is much more than this. Christian mystics have demonstrated time and time again that meditation is completely compatible with Christian belief and reliance on God's grace. Unfortunately, TM is more than just meditation. It includes a set of beliefs about the nature of God and the nature of life that are not Christian beliefs. Christians would do well to avoid Ayurvedic practitioners who promote the TM world view.

In general, Ayurveda probably has less to offer than does TCM. Without the unique therapeutic tool of acupuncture, Ayurveda is just another herbal tradition transmitted through a humoral framework. Though many Ayurvedic herbs will almost certainly prove useful, at this point the available scientific information is less detailed than it is for the herbs used in TCM. The health care consumer should probably wait until Ayurveda has become a bit more "Westernized" before experimenting with its therapies.

Traditional medical systems like Ayurveda and TCM can be quite powerful, but they also have their dangers. Anyone with an interest in these systems should remember that they have almost always been shaped by certain characteristics common to traditional pre-industrial cultures. Traditional cultures emphasize the authority of antiquity rather than of direct experiment. Most importantly, traditional cultures are unitary. Everyone is assumed to share the same set of beliefs, and among those beliefs there is no clear dividing line between religion, philosophy, and science. Christians who wish to experiment with these systems should be careful to select a practitioner who is willing to tease out the useful medical techniques and leave the rest behind.

9

HOMEOPATHY

Homeopathy is endlessly troubling, a collection of paradoxes and contradictions that can frustrate both the skeptical and the sympathetic observer. In the nineteenth century homeopathy competed with conventional medicine so successfully that many physicians anticipated a completely homeopathic future, but today it is farther away from acceptance than almost any other alternative. The scientific evidence for homeopathy is so extensive that a fair-minded inquirer cannot dismiss it, but it is so inconsistent that despite two hundred years of work it does not yet constitute a perfectly convincing demonstration that homeopathy is anything other than a placebo. Homeopathy is a product of the same Western intellectual tradition that produced conventional medicine. In keeping with the highest ideals of that tradition, homeopathy is based on an incisive set of basic principles that rival Newton's laws for elegance and power, but the whole system hinges on a technique of pharmacy that seemingly reduces the medicines to nothing at all.

For all of these reasons and more, this chapter was almost entitled "Why I Wish Homeopathy Didn't Work". No matter what position one takes, homeopathy will eventually prove troubling. A scientific rationalist must eventually wonder why this ridiculous superstition doesn't simply die. Other alternative systems at least offer herbs with mild medicinal activity, or massages that feel good, or diets that lower fat, but this one has only tiny sugar pellets touched by a drop of a solution that once contained an infinitesimal trace of an active ingredient.

How could a medicine that aggressively insists on treating disease with nothing at all survive for over two hundred years?

The advocate has another set of problems. Why hasn't homeopathy triumphed? Hahnemann claimed to have discovered the laws that underlay all true healing. If he was right, then the temporary successes of conventional medicine should long ago have revealed themselves to be an illusion, or even worse, a con game. Hahnemann argued that any attempt to suppress symptoms by chemically inhibiting the body's ability to produce them would inevitably disrupt the body's purposeful response to illness and produce an eventual breakdown of health. In a world full of anti-inflammatories, antihistamines, antacids, and pain-killers, why hasn't this prediction come true? Though the incidence of some chronic diseases has increased, this is almost completely accounted for by the greater number of people living to advanced ages (Manton et al. 2593-2598). Life expectancy continues to go up and infant mortality continues to decline. Why would this be so when most physicians still do not practice according to the Law of Similars?

Even more troubling, why is homeopathy itself so inconsistent in its effectiveness? Not only is this inconsistency characteristic of the scientific evidence concerning homeopathy, it is also typical of homeopathy in practice. Anyone who seriously studies and uses homeopathy will see it succeed brilliantly, sometimes in ways that are almost beyond belief. He or she will also see it fail for no obvious reason at all. The traditional homeopathic response to these failures is to blame them on the prescriber. It can be difficult to find the perfect match between a remedy and the patient's symptoms, but it doesn't seem likely that this is the whole explanation. Sometimes homeopathy just fails, and no one really knows why. Since we don't know why it works, either, this isn't really surprising.

What then are we to do with a discipline like this? There are several possible responses. One is to ignore it completely. Though this is the most comfortable approach, it is hardly the most satisfying. Homeopathy is a true anomaly, and as such it deserves the attention, not the disdain, of the scientific community. The scientific evidence is not yet sufficient to establish homeopathy in the face of the theoretical objections scientists generally raise, but it is certainly extensive enough and consistent enough to be treated as a problem worthy of solution rather than a simple mistake.

There are two general principles which are characteristic of most forms of homeopathy. They are not the only principles proposed by Hahnemann, but they do tend to serve as the common denominator of the several variations of homeopathy found in practice. They also tend to be the focus of most scientific objections to homeopathy.

The first of these is of course the Law of Similars, "let like be cured by like". Substances which produce symptoms in healthy people are capable of curing those same symptoms in sick people. Homeopaths argue that this is the only therapeutic principle which can produce real healing. This definitely rubs conventional physicians the wrong way, but in truth the exclusivity of the claim is the only aspect to which they can object. Though they may not be accustomed to thinking of it as a "law", conventional physicians utilize the principle of similars all the time, whenever they vaccinate, or prescribe any of the several different drugs in common use which were first utilized by homeopaths.

The second principle, the Law of the Minimum Dose, is more problematic. At first it just seems like good sense. Medications should be given in the smallest possible dose which will elicit a healing response, and this response should be allowed to run its course before another dose is given. Who could object to that? In practice, however, Hahnemann's experiments with the minimum dose led directly to the technique of serial dilution which he called potentization. To recall, homeopathic remedies are prepared by diluting the active ingredient in a water and alcohol medium, usually in a ratio of one part active ingredient to either ten or one hundred parts carrier medium. This mixture is then vigorously agitated, and a small amount is removed to serve as the active ingredient in another round of dilution. This process is repeated many times. The medicine is believed to become more and more potent as less and less of the active ingredient is physically present.

For two hundred years, conventional physicians have been grinding out tracts that belittle homeopathic pharmacy in various amusing ways. No one, including the homeopaths, denies that the dilution process proceeds to a point where there is no longer any of the original medicinal substance present. Homeopaths allude to this in a back-handed way when they refer to low potency (meaning less diluted) remedies as "molecular doses". What homeopaths do insist on is that the remedies continue to act, and that this can be demonstrated.

This assertion is usually greeted with the standard "Well, that's just stupid" objection. As previously noted, this is not a convincing refutation. Many truths appear wrong or even silly at first. Common sense would never tell us that an electron can be both a particle and a wave at the same time, or that there are three persons in one God. Yet both of these things are true. We need real evidence to reject the homeopathic claim, not a simple assertion.

At the same time, we cannot be expected to carefully test and analyze every possible truth claim. It is reasonable to limit our efforts to just those propositions which seem to have some chance of proving to be true. All of us sift through truth claims using our knowledge and past experience to sort out those which seem reasonable from those which are simply absurd. In the same way that I don't believe in fairies even though I haven't prowled the woods in night-vision gear to look for them, most scientists assume that homeopathic remedies have no more physiological activity than sugar pills.

This may be reasonable and understandable, but in the case of homeopathy the best available evidence indicates that it is wrong. Unfortunately, most scientists aren't familiar with the best available evidence. Because of its controversial nature, most research on homeopathy has either been ignored or relegated to the homeopathic ghetto where most mainstream scientists and doctors never see it.

Despite these difficulties, there is an increasingly large body of experimental evidence indicating that homeopathic remedies do have measurable effects at least some of the time. Much of the clinical research was summarized by the British Medical Journal in 1991 (Kleijnen et al. 316-323). As discussed in chapter one, the authors of this review article reached reluctantly positive conclusions about homeopathy's efficacy. Since that time, several additional good trials have been published. David Reilly has repeatedly replicated his work on the homeopathic treatment of asthma (Reilly 1601-1606). Jennifer Jacobs has published a study of the successful use of homeopathic remedies to treat childhood diarrhea (Jacobs 719-725). Recently, a large meta-analysis appeared in the Lancet which used statistical techniques to combine the results of many smaller trials to gain statistical power. This meta-analysis confirmed that homeopathy has activity beyond that of placebos (Linde et al. 834-843).

In addition to this clinical work with patients, there is a long history of laboratory research demonstrating an effect of potentized remedies on such test systems as plant growth or enzyme activity in a test tube (Coulter 54-63). This kind of research has been conducted for many decades, but it has only rarely been published in mainstream journals. Together with the clinical research, this body of work constitutes a convincing demonstration of the homeopathic claim.

Except, of course, that it doesn't always work. Right next to the successful trials are other studies that show that homeopathic remedies are no more effective than placebo. Many physicians have a vague impression that these negative trials are the majority, and that the positive trials are few in number and are therefore probably the result of random chance. This is emphatically not the case. The real situation is more complicated and less explicable.

Most careful studies show an effect of homeopathy. The more careful the study, the more likely it is to show an effect. But, a higher proportion of trials fail than would be typical if a more conventional therapy was tested in the same way. Homeopathic remedies are active, but in a less predictable, less consistent way than ordinary drugs. So far, the research doesn't point to an explanation. We don't know why homeopathy works the way it does.

This means that homeopathy can't be ignored but it also isn't a fully mature therapy, despite its two hundred year history. At this point we don't know what its limits are, or when it can be expected to work. We don't know the illnesses it is most capable of treating.

One possible answer comes from homeopathy itself. Homeopaths resist the idea of specific illnesses, what they call "disease entities". Rather than focusing on characteristics which allow the same disease to be identified in different patients, homeopaths prefer to focus on those unique symptoms which distinguish a particular patient's pattern of resistance to disease. In its most extreme form, this approach can ignore common disease symptoms altogether, in favor of finding a remedy which expresses a patient's "essence".

This approach has come to be known as classical homeopathy, though it is practiced by a minority of homeopaths and wasn't emphasized by Hahnemann himself. A better term is probably constitutional homeopathy, since this is more purely descriptive and less likely to exclude those practitioners who might prescribe a constitutional remedy on occasion but who are also willing to prescribe on the basis of more limited disease symptoms.

Constitutional homeopathy is the clearest example of the assumptions homeopaths bring to the debate. If the remedies are inconsistent, they argue, it is because people are inconsistent. Homeopathy doesn't act through the biochemical channels used by conventional drugs. It provides information only, and the patient's body does the healing on the basis of that information. Since homeopathy relies on the patient's own recuperative powers, it will inevitably provide more erratic results than chemical agents which act directly against disease.

This is an intriguing hypothesis, but at this point it remains a hypothesis. We don't know how information is encoded in the remedies or how the body receives the information. If these details could be filled in, then the orthodox scientific community would need to take this hypothesis seriously. It is certainly consistent with the clinical experience accumulated by homeopaths over the last two centuries.

If the hypothesis was confirmed, then despite its occasionally erratic performance homeopathy would prove to be a tool of astonishing usefulness. Many illnesses are not the result of a direct attack by some outside agent. They are instead a regulatory failure. The subtle interlocking mechanisms which the body uses to control and organize its functions don't always operate with perfect efficiency. Sometimes they overreact slightly, or underreact a bit, or maybe they just drift a little. However it happens, we find our immune systems reacting to harmless pollen, or the inflammatory mechanisms which should protect us staying activated long enough to actually damage the sensitive cartilage in our joints.

Conventional drugs don't correct this failure of homeostatic control. They override it. This is better than nothing, but it tends to bring with it a slew of side-effects and unintended consequences.

Homeopathy hints at a way to tune the homeostatic mechanisms directly. As discussed in the previous chapter, acupuncture also promises this kind of control, but needles are clearly more invasive than the little pills of homeopathy. In addition, practitioners who have used both therapies indicate that acupuncture tends to impose its own "setting" on the body's controls. In contrast, homeopathy does nothing more than provide feedback of the body's current state so that it can adjust itself to a more effective level of functioning. If we believe that God's creation can be trusted, then no therapy trusts the body more than homeopathy.

Given the potential value of the payoff, serious research into homeopathy is a worthy gamble. It is irresponsible of the scientific community to discourage rather than encourage this research, but that is in fact the most common reaction. The argument with homeopathy is an old one, and the scars run deep.

Surely the time has come to acknowledge that homeopathy can consistently produce anomalous results, and that we need to understand how and why. There is almost certainly a physical mechanism involved which the tools of science can reveal. To accomplish this, however, those tools will need to be focused on the task of understanding homeopathy rather than debunking it. There is a sufficient body of evidence to establish that debunking will not succeed.

This kind of research is also necessary to address the lingering doubts held by some Christians. Until the physical mechanism is fully understood, there are those who will continue to wonder if homeopathy is a variety of occultism. Once we can convincingly explain the homeopathic effect in purely natural terms, then those doubts should disappear.

Unfortunately, as with so many other alternatives, the research has not yet been done. We are forced to make our decision on what is admittedly preliminary information. In the case of homeopathy, an argument can be made for utilizing the remedies under certain circumstances despite our incomplete understanding.

Theologically based scruples seem unwarranted. When a pharmaceutical procedure which involves nothing more arcane than mixing and shaking consistently produces results, then the most parsimonious, as well as obvious, explanation is that a physical process is responsible. Mystery does not equal evil.

When we lack complete information about a therapy's mechanism of action, it is reasonable to consider the possibility of an unanticipated toxic effect emerging at some point in the future. This seems unlikely with homeopathy. The one thing that both advocates and opponents agree on is that the remedies are safe. Opponents believe that they are nothing more than sugar pills, while advocates argue that only someone who needs a given remedy will react to it. Whatever one's preconceptions, it is hard to see how the incredibly dilute preparations characteristic of homeopathy could cause harm.

We also have the clinical experience of homeopaths to draw on, and they have left a very reassuring record of safety. It is important to remember that for most of its history homeopathy has been practiced by well educated professional physicians, indistinguishable from their more conventional colleagues in every way except for their choice of therapy. These physicians were trained in (and indeed, helped to shape) the Western scientific tradition. Their observations constitute a more reliable body of evidence than the ad hoc anecdotes which we have for other alternatives. Two hundred years of experience teach us that the remedies are nontoxic. The only real danger is that the wrong remedy will be selected and will fail to act.

Since this is a real possibility, homeopathy should only be used for mild, self-limited conditions. It simply isn't reliable enough for serious illness or emergencies. Though it can be used as an adjunct in these cases, homeopathy should only be used while conventional care is being sought. As a good rule of thumb, one should only use homeopathy in those conditions which one would feel comfortable treating with symptom relieving over-the-counter drugs. If a little voice tells you to see a doctor, see a doctor.

There are more subtle hazards associated with homeopathy, but they tend to be limited to people whose study of and involvement in homeopathy is much deeper than the typical self-care user. They are hazards of attitude, not physical health. Serious students of homeopathy, steeped in homeopathic thought, are sometimes aggressive defenders of homeopathy's exclusivity. Samuel Hahnemann had no interest in founding yet another medical sect. He wanted to discover the natural laws that allowed any and all medicine to stimulate healing. Some people believe that he succeeded.

Those people who are convinced that the Hahnemannian system is a complete, fully satisfactory solution to the problem of health and healing tend to be much less accepting of other medical systems than is common in the alternative world. If a therapy isn't based on the Law of Similars, then hard core Hahnemannians consider it suppressive and dangerous. In practice, this means that these homeopaths not only reject most conventional medicine, they reject most non-homeopathic alternative medicine as well. If homeopathy doesn't get you well, then either you didn't do it right or you are incurable.

Apologists for conventional medicine often argue that this is a danger throughout the alternative community. They paint grim pictures of cancer patients wasting away while treating themselves with bizarre remedies prescribed by charismatic quacks. In this vision, Svengali-like alternative practitioners draw gullible patients away from the good and decent regular doctors who could cure them.

While this does occasionally happen, it is quite rare. The nature of the alternative community generally precludes it. Since alternative therapies are by definition non-mainstream, they are usually not a patient's first recourse. Most people seek out an alternative practitioner after a conventional physician has failed to give them relief. Once they have found an alternative they usually add this to their conventional treatment rather than discontinuing the old in favor of the new (Astin 1548-1553). This is normally quite acceptable to alternative practitioners, since they commonly share a commitment to the value of multiple points of view.

Classical homeopaths can be the exception to this rule. Homeopathy sometimes attracts fervent ideologues who find the idea of inviolable universal laws of healing powerfully appealing. Homeopaths of this stripe can be quite rigid in their insistence on sola similia—homeopathic healing only.

Our knowledge of homeopathy is not yet deep enough to make this a defensible position. Hahnemann's system is a set of scientific hypotheses, not a revelation from God. As such, it requires verification. Even if homeopathy were to be completely verified, this would not invalidate the body of knowledge accumulated by conventional medicine, though it might lead us to reassess the long-term effect of some conventional therapies. Suppressive therapies would still have applications, however, because much of what these therapies suppress is simple suffering. As anyone who has suffered knows, relief from suffering is worth some cost. No one should be made to feel guilty about pursuing that relief.

Homeopathy can also foster an unhealthy degree of self-absorption. In constitutional homeopathy, anything and everything can be a symptom pointing towards one's constitutional type. If one is working with a professional homeopath, then one is less likely to slip into the game of "what's my type", but it is a real danger for people studying on their own. There is nothing wrong with wanting to understand oneself, but this should not be our primary focus. Christians should turn their thoughts upward and outward rather than inward.

Finding one's constitutional type also requires that one "medicalize" one's character flaws. Our sins become symptoms, with no significance other than to point to the proper remedy. While it is perfectly appropriate and necessary for a physician to suspend all moral judgements when treating a patient, it is less justifiable to adopt this attitude in regard to oneself. We are to repent of our sins, not cherish them as a pointer to our deepest self.

For most of us, though, these are not likely hazards. Most of us can safely take advantage of homeopathy's strengths. How do we do this?

If we want constitutional treatment, we should seek out a qualified M.D. who practices homeopathically. Not only is this the safest approach, but we will probably get better results than if we attempted to treat ourselves or have ourselves treated by a friend or acquaintance. A physician's greater objectivity will usually result in more accurate prescribing.

In self-care situations, there are several possible approaches. The simplest is to purchase one of the widely available combination formulas for our condition and take it according to the label instructions. Combination formulas contain several remedies whose symptom pictures will cover most people suffering from a given condition. Because they combine remedies in this way, it isn't necessary to search through the available possibilities to find the single remedy which matches. This dramatically simplifies the process of using homeopathy.

Traditional homeopaths have always objected to combination formulas, but their reservations have little relevance to most of us. Hahnemann, reacting to the incredibly complex prescriptions utilized by the conventional physicians of his day, made it a tenet of his "new school" that only one remedy should be given at a time. His primary concern was that the physician be able to clearly interpret the success or failure of a given prescription without the additional complication of trying to figure out which ingredient actually did the work. In addition, homeopaths have long argued that the deepest, most profound healing can only occur with the use of the single remedy in high (meaning more dilute) potency.

These may be legitimate protocols for professional practitioners doing constitutional prescribing, though even here the emphasis on the single remedy seems more like a rule of thumb than an inviolable law. Most of us, though, aren't doing constitutional prescribing. We don't care which ingredients did the work as long as we feel better. We aren't trying to achieve perfect health, we are just trying to get through this cold or this sore throat. Combination formulas work superbly for these purposes.

We can stay at this point indefinitely if we wish, adding homeopathic combination formulas to our repertoire of home remedies without any additional knowledge of homeopathy being necessary at all. If, however, we wish to go beyond this to the use of single remedies some study will be necessary. Homeopathy works if we match the symptom picture correctly, and it fails if we don't, so knowing the symptom pictures of the remedies is crucial. This doesn't necessarily mean memorization, but one should at least have a passing familiarity with a good homeopathic self-care handbook before attempting to prescribe "under the gun" of an active acute illness. Once we have some background knowledge, a basic home kit of twenty to thirty remedies will allow us to treat most minor illnesses with a fair degree of success.

Homeopathy isn't perfect. It can be maddeningly unpredictable. Its practitioners can be infuriatingly unyielding in their insistence that the rest of the world return to the One True Medicine. Nonetheless, out of all the various therapies available in the alternative community, homeopathy seems most likely to offer something really new to medicine. If conventional physicians and researchers could be persuaded to give homeopathy the examination it deserves, the mystery of homeopathy would almost certainly illuminate the deeper mystery of healing itself.

10

CHIROPRACTIC

Chiropractic is a bit of a chameleon. At times, chiropractic looks like just another specialized branch of conventional medicine. Chiropractors are addressed as "doctor", their offices look like doctors' offices, and one can even get insurance reimbursement for their services. Just when one has grown comfortable thinking of them as "back doctors", a smiling chiropractor will produce a chart showing how a variety of apparently unrelated diseases are *really* caused by subluxations, or misalignments, of the spine.

This odd duality is fundamental to chiropractic's identity. It is the only alternative which has achieved a degree of institutional acceptance while preserving its alternative perspective. Chiropractors have successfully sold themselves as the medical professionals best equipped to handle musculo-skeletal problems of the back, while also maintaining their allegiance to the idea that the spine is the most crucial organ of the human body in the genesis of disease.

It isn't surprising that this strikes some people as just a bit shifty. Sometimes chiropractors plaintively insist that all they want is to be accepted. At other times, they talk as if their real goal is to completely dethrone M.D.s as monarchs of the health care system and put D.C.s in their place. Different chiropractors will emphasize one or the other of these poles. Sometimes the same chiropractor will flip back and forth, or even insist on both at the same time. This makes choosing a chiropractor an uncertain process for anyone who just wants relief of back pain.

The perception of shiftiness is not enhanced by chiropractors' willingness to utilize hard sell techniques to bring in patients. Chiropractors frequently run contests and promotions in which the prize is a free chiropractic exam. As has often been pointed out, chiropractors never met a spine they couldn't improve (Weil 132-133), so a free exam usually results in a new patient.

To be fair, some of this is a product of cultural and class differences between M.D.s and D.C.s, rather than a deliberate attempt to defraud. Historians have noted that chiropractors have tended to settle in rural areas and in other areas that are underserved by physicians (J.S. Moore 119). Chiropractic education has always been both cheaper and easier than conventional medical education. Though the gap has narrowed in recent years, no one would argue that even the best chiropractic education available is the equivalent of Johns Hopkins or Harvard Medical School. Once they graduate, M.D.s (despite much recent whining) can count on a comfortable income and social prestige. Chiropractors are always just on the edge of respectability, and if they achieve a large income they do it by drive and salesmanship.

In short, M.D.s are among our culture's elite; honored, respected, and rewarded in every way our culture can provide. Chiropractors are members of a scrappy profession which has fought for its place on the margins. Chiropractic came along just as conventional medicine was consolidating its grip on the culture, and chiropractic survived only because of the bulldog tenacity of the D.C.s. If chiropractors are aggressive, they have had to be. If they tend to bob and weave, sounding conciliatory and conventional at times only to assert their alternative commitments at surprising moments, then we should remember that this ability to duck from one shelter to another has been one of the secrets of their survival.

Unfortunately, chiropractors have had very little interest in proving the value of their therapy to their arch rivals, the M.D.s. M.D.s have been just as reluctant to examine a system which they have generally regarded as the epitome of quackery. As a result, we have very little real knowledge of what chiropractic can actually accomplish.

There is growing consensus that it is at least as effective as conventional medicine in the treatment of uncomplicated back pain. Several good studies have demonstrated that chiropractors normally get people back to work quicker than M.D.s, and that patients prefer chiropractic (Carey et al. 913-917). M.D.s have grumbled that patient satisfaction can be affected by a variety of factors other than the success of treatment, such as the physical contact required to perform a chiropractic adjustment, or the chiropractor's willingness to provide an explanation for the patient's pain. As a patient, these objections strike me as sour grapes. Rather than disparaging these aspects of chiropractic care, one would hope that conventional physicians would also see fit to incorporate touch and communication into their practices.

It is true that studies of chiropractic cannot be double-blinded because of the nature of the therapy. Both practitioner and patient know when an adjustment has been performed. Nonetheless, there seems to be no compelling reason to doubt these studies. When conventional medicine and chiropractic go head to head, the cultural authority of M.D.s provides some real advantages in producing a potent placebo effect. Despite this, the chiropractors continue to succeed.

It is also worth pointing out that accusations of a placebo effect cut both ways. Studies have consistently shown that chiropractors produce results equal to or better than conventional physicians. If the chiropractic success is purely the product of the placebo effect, what does this say about the ability of conventional medicine to treat back pain? It is a foundational assumption of the controlled trial that a therapy which produces effects equivalent to placebo is no more than a placebo itself. If chiropractic is inactive in the treatment of uncomplicated back pain, then so is conventional medicine.

It seems more reasonable to assume that both disciplines have some power to effect the course of a bout with back pain. This is certainly what patients report. The patient's own experience is the most important standard for the success of back pain treatment, since the overwhelming majority of patients do not have a serious illness causing their pain. All they have is pain, and any therapy which can relieve it is a successful therapy.

When two therapies are clearly equivalent in their ability to relieve suffering, then we must make our decision about which to use on the basis of other factors. Safety is obviously a central concern, and many past attacks on chiropractic have focused on the supposed hazards of the chiropractic adjustment. As typically performed, an adjustment is quick and produces a cracking noise which is quite dramatic if one is not anticipating it. It is not unreasonable to wonder if this procedure is entirely safe.

Enough information now exists to assess the degree of hazard from an adjustment with a fair degree of accuracy. The chief danger seems to be stroke induced by the rapid flexion of the blood vessels in the neck. Serious complications like this occur between five and ten times in every ten million adjustments (Hurwitz et al. 1746-1759)

This can be compared to the hazards of drug treatment, the primary therapeutic option of the conventional physician. Nonsteroidal anti-inflammatory drugs such as ibuprofen are commonly prescribed for back pain. These drugs are known to frequently damage the gastrointestinal tract of patients who take them long-term, sometimes producing life threatening bleeding ulcers. It has been estimated that up to 20,000 deaths a year result from this complication (Wolfe 37-44, 47-48).

Complications from chiropractic are much less common. It is probable that serious drug reactions outnumber chiropractic complications several hundred times over (Dabbs and Lauretti 530-536). There are new anti-inflammatory medications in development that may be significantly safer, but these medications have no track record as yet. Chiropractic has been in use for over a century. It seems clear that chiropractic is the safer therapy.

Though this calculation is relatively straightforward, the issue becomes more ambiguous when we look beyond back pain. When the effectiveness of a therapy for a given condition is unclear, then the hazards of the therapy have to be added to the potential hazard of the disease itself if the treatment fails to halt or correct it. Chiropractors often argue that their therapy is generally useful for a variety of conditions, and here the evidence is much less clear.

The chiropractic position is not, however, wholly irrational. There are small studies indicating that chiropractic may produce improvement in headaches, painful menstruation, and bedwetting (Fugh-Berman 57-59). None of these studies is large enough to be conclusive, but it is striking that the results exist at all. Perhaps the chiropractors are onto something when they suggest that an organ's function can be affected by mechanical interference with the nerves leading to it.

It would be a mistake, however, to jump from this to the full-blown chiropractic position that this kind of interference is the primary influence on human health. There is essentially no evidence to support this assertion, and a great deal of evidence that contradicts it. In many ways the chiropractic assertion more closely resembles a piece of religious doctrine than a scientific hypothesis, stemming as it does from the philosophy of chiropractic's founder and his son.

D.D. Palmer, the first chiropractor, and his son B.J., explained chiropractic's mechanism of action in terms that were as spiritual or mystical as they were physiological. They described the body's functioning as organized by Innate Intelligence, often referred to simply as "Innate". Innate is the manifestation in the individual of Universal Intelligence, which permeates and organizes the universe. Innate, roughly equivalent to chi or life force, controls the body through the nervous system. If there is no interference with Innate, it will coordinate the body in the most harmonious possible way, producing a state of superb natural health.

Since Innate will always produce the best possible response to an attack on the body's integrity, in the chiropractic view a failure to heal can almost always be traced back to some interference with the activity of Innate. Since Innate utilizes the nervous system, health problems result from a disruption of the nervous system's coordinating function, usually by a physical impingement on the nerves as they emerge from the spine. This can be corrected by the chiropractic adjustment, allowing Innate to restore health.

This isn't quite science, but it isn't exactly religion either. It sits uneasily between the two, straddling the divide in a way that isn't satisfying to either the conventional scientist or the careful theologian. It resembles the Chinese view of life as process and pattern, wedded to a somewhat oversimplified version of Western physiology.

Since this scheme is intended to address issues of physical health, it is perhaps understandable that it doesn't consider sin or salvation. Unfortunately, health and illness cannot be fully understood without them. In chiropractic philosophy, ill health is the result of an accidental disruption, and the body's normal state is harmonious and perfect. There is no room in this scheme for an assault on the body that the body cannot counter or control.

Christians know that the harmony of creation has been deeply disrupted. "We know that the whole creation has been groaning in labor pains until now," (Romans 8:22). The world is fallen, and the fall brought with it sickness and death. There is more wrong with us than misaligned spines.

Chiropractic is clearly incomplete, both as an explanation of and a solution to ill-health. Being incomplete is not, however, the same thing as being flat out wrong. Some critics have accused chiropractic of creeping paganism, based on the chiropractic willingness to utilize quasi-spiritual but non-Christian terminology (Sneed and Sneed 92-93).

This critique seems far too strong. Chiropractic makes no attempt to influence any spiritual force or entity directly. Instead, it works only with the material channels by which the physical body is controlled. A

Christian neurologist who believed in the presence of the soul could describe his or her work in the same way.

The vast majority of chiropractors treat chiropractic as a holistically oriented medical discipline which is friendly to spiritual perspectives, not as a religion in itself. If chiropractic isn't asking ultimate questions, then we can't fault it for not providing Christian answers.

Indeed, even though the terms are not Christian, much of chiropractic philosophy is quite compatible with Christianity. Though God is transcendent, he is also immanent in creation, and creation reveals much of the Creator. The magnificently complex and adaptive human body is one of the clearest signs of God's design. "Innate Intelligence" is not a bad way to describe how the body mirrors the radiant Reason of the Lord. We can hardly accuse chiropractors of occultism or paganism simply because they regard the body as suffused by spirit, since this is an assumption chiropractic shares with Christianity.

Chiropractic philosophy is only dangerous if it is regarded as a completely sufficient answer to both our medical and our spiritual needs. Chiropractors may occasionally argue that chiropractic could take the place of modern medicine, but no responsible chiropractor would assert that it could replace religion as well. Though chiropractors are often guilty of overselling their therapy, they don't normally claim that it can provide freedom from death or salvation from sin.

Their medical claims are exaggerated enough, however. There is no medical evidence to support the universal efficacy of chiropractic. Since chiropractic philosophy is insufficient to explain the world's evil (even when limited to that evil which manifests as human illness), chiropractic claims cannot be justified philosophically either.

This can help us make decisions as patients. Chiropractic is a safe and effective treatment for musculoskeletal problems, especially back pain. It is effective enough for headache that it can often serve as a primary treatment for this condition as well, as long as a more serious cause has been ruled out by medical exam. Beyond this, chiropractic should serve as an adjunct therapy only. And there is *no* justification for healthy people with no symptoms to receive regular adjustments.

Chiropractors often argue that everyone should receive regular chiropractic care as a form of health maintenance, just as one receives regular dental exams. The difference between these two is that dental neglect has clear consequences, whereas chiropractors have never demonstrated that spinal misalignments result in later disease. This is an interesting hypothesis, and it would be good to see someone attempt to prove or disprove it, but at this point the work has not been done. It is not reasonable to expect people to submit themselves on a regular basis to a procedure which has real risks, however small, just because it seems like a good idea. Some more definitive evidence is necessary before chiropractic can be considered a preventive health measure.

As a patient, we should select a chiropractor who is willing to allow us to make the decisions about when we need to be adjusted. Not all chiropractors practice in this way. Some require that you sign a contract committing to a pre-set course of treatment. Others will only accept patients who "really understand chiropractic". This normally means patients who are willing to receive regular adjustments for a lifetime for "health maintenance". Neither of these models is acceptable. Until the chiropractors prove their case, adjustments should be used for symptom relief only. The patient is always the best judge of his or her symptoms.

Some conventionally minded consumer advocates go even further. They suggest that patients use only those chiropractors who have repudiated the monocausal theory of disease and who limit their practice to back and neck pain. Though this sounds reasonable and conservative, this standard almost completely eliminates chiropractic as an option for most of us, since chiropractors who practice this way are few and far between. Chiropractic is still very much an alternative, and most chiropractors are proud of their alternative perspective. They aren't about to abandon it to become glorified physical therapists under the control of M.D.s.

This is O.K. If chiropractors are given to exaggerating their ability to heal, conventional physicians unfairly belittle it, for reasons that can only be described as self-serving. If the price for pain relief is a little chiropractic bombast and bluster, most of us can tolerate that. As long as we retain the right to make decisions about our care, then we can make those decisions with a more realistic view of chiropractic's power.

In many ways the chiropractor's skill is a more important criteria than his philosophy. Like all manual arts, adjustments can be done well or poorly. When it's my back being cracked, I want good hands doing the cracking. This can often be determined by talking to current and former patients. If a chiropractor has good hands and is willing to let patients make their own decisions, then an exaggerated faith in the power of chiropractic is excusable. We should not, however, accept a chiropractor who insists that we share this belief and use only chiropractic health care, or even use chiropractic as a first recourse for non-musculoskeletal complaints.

Despite their claims, chiropractors cannot serve as primary health care providers in the way M.D.s can. D.C.s are insufficiently trained in the art of differential diagnosis. They are all too willing to treat everything that comes their way with spinal adjustments. They are often reluctant to refer patients to more conventional practitioners (though to be fair, this reluctance runs both ways).

Even given all this, we must not lose sight of the fact that chiropractors possess a powerful, drug-free way of treating debilitating aches and pains. Chiropractors can provide real relief of suffering. We shouldn't hesitate to take advantage of this, though we may want to keep one hand on our wallet while we do so.

11

THE ALTERNATIVE LION'S DEN

Alternative medicine unquestionably demands more of the patient than does conventional medicine. This isn't because alternative medicine focuses more on lifestyle change, though this is frequently the case. It is because alternative medicine has real hazards in addition to real benefits, and one must avoid the hazards to reap the benefits.

If we would prefer to place our trust in a medical authority figure and leave the decision making to them, then alternative medicine is not for us. If we are uncomfortable weighing risk against benefit when both are only imperfectly known, then alternative medicine is not for us. If we don't feel up to the task of working our way through medical literature to assess and evaluate evidence for ourselves, then alternative medicine is not for us. Conventional medicine is unquestionably the most effective medicine yet devised by human beings, and it can take good care of us for a lifetime.

But—conventional medicine is more a blunt instrument than a rapier. It is prone to the production of side effects, and it isn't very good at handling chronic conditions in a way which can be tolerated by the patient. Worst of all, the conventional medical community is deeply committed to materialism. Although there are many fine Christian physicians, no top flight medical journal would ever publish an article which was explicitly Christian in its assumptions.

Alternative medicine can correct some of these deficiencies, but only if we can avoid some traps along the way. There really is such a thing as a quack, and there really are con men willing to take money from the desperate. We must also remember that though holistic practitioners frequently claim to be friendly to spiritual perspectives, this acceptance often does not extend to Christianity. Although the principles for discernment outlined in Chapter Four can help us locate therapies which might be useful, it is worth summarizing some more cautionary guidelines which can help us avoid the worst abuses.

Principle Number One: There are no miracle cures.

Alternative medicine is full of useful techniques and useful therapies. There are even people around for whom one or more of these therapies may have tilted the balance from death to life. But, in general, there are *no* conditions for which alternative medicine offers a cure unavailable through conventional medicine. Alternative medicine is good at strengthening people, not curing diseases. It almost always works best as an adjunct to conventional therapy, not a replacement. If someone tells you that he has a secret cure for cancer, or multiple sclerosis, or anything else, he is either mistaken or lying (and unfortunately, he's probably lying).

Principle Number Two: Avoid exclusive claims.

If someone insists that they possess the only true path to health, they are wrong. If they want us to abandon all therapies but their's, they are guilty of the same arrogance which allows conventional physicians to casually dismiss any medicine but their own. Since conventional medicine can make a stronger case for exclusivity than any other system, if we won't accept this from regular M.D.s we certainly should not accept it from an alternative practitioner. It is a strength of alternative medicine that it contains a variety of potentially useful therapies. We should not surrender this advantage.

Principle Number Three: Avoid mysterious machines.

Con men love impressive electronic gadgetry. Blinking lights and moving dials look uniquely powerful and scientific. If someone offers to treat you or diagnose you with a miracle machine unknown to modern science, run. With only two possible exceptions, there are no alternative devices with enough evidence to justify their use.

The first exception is biofeedback equipment when used by a licensed clinical psychologist. Though not all applications of biofeedback have proven equally sound, it can be helpful for a variety of stress related conditions. It may not, however, have any compelling advantages over simpler stress reduction techniques—like prayer.

The remaining exception requires more caution. This is the use of electro-stimulation of acupuncture points. Though this is probably a useful extension of traditional practice, there are other electronic devices in use by acupuncturists that are less defensible. In particular, the use of "energy" measurements at acupuncture points for diagnostic purposes is not supported by either the scientific literature or Traditional Chinese Medicine.

Principle Number Four: Avoid invasive procedures unless performed by a conventional physician.

An invasive procedure is one in which a foreign object of some kind is inserted into the body, either through the skin or through a body orifice. This can be anything from an I.V. to an enema to surgery. Any time something is introduced into the body, there is a danger of injury or infection. If a drug is introduced as well, many of the body's normal defenses against toxins are bypassed. Whatever the drug is, it will almost always achieve a higher concentration in the bloodstream when it is given by I.V. or injection rather than orally. The margin for error is much smaller.

Conventional medicine possesses a superb set of techniques and protocols for handling the dangers of invasive procedures. Unless they have been conventionally trained, alternative practitioners are generally not well versed in these precautions. I once asked the proprietor of a colon therapy clinic if the nozzles of their colonic machines were sterilized between uses. There was an uncomfortable pause, and then she said, "Well, that's certainly something we'd like to begin doing in the future." In the age of AIDS, it is criminally negligent to insert a medical instrument into multiple rectums without sterilization.

Similarly, there are no alternative agents that I would allow someone to inject into my body. Given the increased level of hazard from this method of administration, I want a drug to be *very* well understood before someone shoots it into me with a needle. Anecdotal evidence is not enough. I want careful studies and a good understanding of a drug's mechanism of action. There are no alternative drugs that can meet this standard.

Principle Number Five: Avoid occultism.

Though this has been previously discussed, it is the most important principle of all and it bears repeating. As Christians, we are forbidden to dabble in the occult. The problem is knowing what is and what is not prohibited. I would adamantly reject any standard that prohibited a therapy simply because it isn't fully understood. The assumption here seems to be that if there is no known natural process at work then it must be supernatural and therefore wrong.

There is an additional category neglected by this scheme, that of unknown natural processes. Anomalous results point us towards what we don't yet know. It isn't evil to probe the unknown. It is the very engine of knowledge.

This having been said, there are still some alternative therapies which are clearly occult. As discussed in Chapter Four, the most obvious are those variations of shamanism or channeling which involve contacting a spirit in some way. It should be clear that this is an unacceptable compromise of our complete reliance on the Lord, but there are practical concerns as well. We have no reason to believe that spirits are uniformly benign. Indeed, some of them are downright dangerous. Toying with spirits is roughly akin to sitting on a lit stick of dynamite in the hope of achieving flight. The hazards seem somewhat more certain than any possible rewards.

Another danger sign is any attempt to influence external reality directly through the application of the will. This is the essence of magic. Few modern practitioners would admit that they are practicing magic, but if an individual is attempting to change something in the outside world by focusing his or her thoughts, it is hard to describe it any other way. Many of the so-called "energy therapies" operate in precisely this fashion. Therapeutic touch and reiki, for instance, may be white magic, but they are magic nonetheless. Avoid them.

Finally, any system that teaches that certain objects have an inherent power to influence the world by their presence alone is tilting in dangerous directions. Crystal healing may utilize holistic health terminology, but it is nothing more than the ancient practice of using gemstones as amulets for good luck. Christians do not wear amulets.

This last criteria is fuzzier than the others, and a degree of judgement is called for. Objects are capable of projecting forms of influence that aren't immediately apparent to the senses, such as radiation or magnetism. Whether or not it is effective, it isn't superstition to believe that magnets might have an effect on arthritis pain. It is superstition to believe that a magnetic lodestone can somehow order circumstances to produce good luck for its owner.

When considering the question of occultism, one should always obey one's own conscience. If you cannot escape the lingering suspicion that some therapy is a form of magic or witchcraft, then heed that voice and abandon that therapy. You may need to ignore some trusted authority to do so, perhaps even the authority of this book. For instance, I do not believe that either vitalism or mystery equals occultism, so I am comfortable with homeopathy and some forms of acupuncture. If you don't find this argument convincing, I would rather you listened to your own inner promptings than accept the judgement of this book when you don't really feel comfortable doing so. Let the Holy Spirit guide you.

If we eliminate all the therapies proscribed by these standards, what are we left with? There are two broad categories of therapies that are simultaneously useful, alternative, and theologically acceptable. The first consists of alternative systems with a long history of use, so that the accumulated experience of patients can give us a good sense of the potential risks and benefits. From a theological standpoint, the best systems are those which are open to spiritual reality, but which do not directly address spiritual issues themselves. Herbalism, homeopathy, and chiropractic fall into this category. The scientific evidence for homeopathy and chiropractic isn't perfect, but they have been around long enough that we can be reasonably sure they are safe. There are so many forms of herbalism that it is hard to generalize about them, but there are certainly individual herbs from many traditions that are both safe and effective.

Traditional Chinese Medicine is somewhat more problematic. It contains both effective and ineffective therapies, but traditional practitioners don't normally discriminate between them. Theologically, the boundaries between TCM and Chinese religion and philosophy are sometimes fuzzy. They can be distinguished, but a traditional practitioner may have no interest in doing so. The safest approach to TCM is to find a medical acupuncturist who can apply useful Chinese techniques within the context of Western medicine.

The second broad category of therapies worth consideration might be termed new science. These are the therapeutic applications of our growing understanding of the health effects of various lifestyle factors, especially diet and exercise. Dietary supplements also fall into this category. These interventions are normally considered more conservative than the first group. Conventional physicians are more comfortable with them, since they fit better with the rest of Western science.

This does not necessarily mean that the scientific evidence for these therapies is better. It is generally impossible to run a true double-blind trial for dietary changes and exercise, because the subject always knows if the intervention is being used or not. It is easier to run conclusive trials for dietary supplements, but many potentially useful nutrients have yet to be carefully studied.

Despite these difficulties in experimental design and the scandalous lack of scientific attention, many nutritional and exercise recommendations have been around long enough to demonstrate their safety. None of them have been incontrovertibly proven effective, but they are generally safe and likely to be of benefit. We can use them with a clear conscience, since there are essentially no theological objections to their use.

None of the therapies in either group, taken separately or together, is capable of replacing conventional medicine. The corpus of conventional medicine is one of the greatest intellectual achievements of the human race. The medicine of the next century will be a recognizable descendent of the conventional medicine of today.

Nonetheless, it seems likely that at least some perspectives that are currently considered alternative will be integrated into twenty first century medicine. Alternative medicine is capable of adding such a useful degree of flexibility to medicine that it would be outrageous if it was ignored. The gentle, subtle remedies characteristic of alternative medicine augment conventional therapeutics at precisely its weakest point.

Conventional medicine is superb crisis medicine, but not everything is a crisis. In a crisis it is appropriate to take over for a body that has been stretched beyond its limits. The body's control systems can be overridden to produce a more effective response. Functions can be sustained through artificial supports. If necessary, vital organs can even be temporarily taken "offline" to allow for surgical repair. Modern medicine is capable of truly astonishing feats.

But not all medical problems call for this kind of intervention. Sometimes these interventions can even be counter-productive. Human beings are adaptive, feedback responsive wholes. Any intervention will produce a response. We cannot adjust our physiology as if we were turning the tuning knob on a radio, because this particular radio has its own ideas about the proper station to receive. If we attempt to change the body's response by brute force, we will be met with quirky, unforseen reactions and side effects.

Alternative medicine is generally better than conventional medicine at guiding the body rather than forcing it. In the event of serious illness, this may mean that none of the common alternatives will be potent enough to do the job. If, however, we have one of the troubling, but not life threatening conditions that constitute ninety percent of the human race's medical complaints, then alternative medicine may provide us with a gentle way to coax our bodies back to homeostasis. It is even possible that these mild corrections may help prevent more dangerous perturbations in our health in the future.

As health care consumers, we can take advantage of these capabilities now. To do this, we will need to reorient our usual approach to health care. Most of us begin with our conventional physician and only experiment with alternatives if we fail to get relief. Most of the problems brought to M.D.s are either self-limited or stress related (Virji 22-26). Since there is no clear cure for these kinds of illnesses, physicians typically provide symptomatic treatment. The patient is made more comfortable but the cause of his or her illness is not affected.

These are precisely the kinds of conditions that alternative medicine can treat effectively. If the patient is suffering from a mild viral infection, then tincture of echinacea can strengthen immune response and shorten the illness. If someone has been sidelined by a musculoskeletal complaint which is painful but not dangerous, then acupuncture or chiropractic can restore mobility without the hazards of pharmaceutical muscle relaxers or anti-inflammatories. Homeopathy can provide at least some relief for almost any condition which is not life threatening. These remedies should be used first, before we turn to powerful drugs or surgery.

If there is any doubt in our mind about the seriousness of our condition, then we should immediately see an M.D. for diagnostic purposes. But, if the doctor offers us only symptom-masking drugs for comfort's sake, we should immediately turn to a more productive alternative therapy. This is what alternative medicine does best.

We should also allow conventional medicine to do what it does best. There is no medical system that handles serious illness as well as conventional medicine. If we have cancer, or heart disease, or a life-threatening infection, there is no one who stands a better chance of curing us than a regular M.D. We may want to take herbs or vitamins as adjuncts, but our primary therapy should be one developed and tested with all the tools of Western science.

If we do learn to rely on alternative medicine for minor complaints, there is one more pitfall we should be aware of. It isn't a hazard of the therapies. It is a vulnerability that some of us are subject to as patients. Some of us are prone to experiencing a wide variety of physical symptoms when we are under psychological stress. We may have headaches, or backaches, or irritable bowel syndrome, or a variety of other possible complaints. We are not imagining these conditions, or making them up. They are real physical problems, caused by our nervous system's tendency to translate psychological distress into physical tension.

Physicians call this somaticizing. Regular medicine doesn't offer very good solutions for these kinds of problems, so somaticizers are often driven to seek relief through alternative medicine. Unfortunately, even though alternative medicine can temporarily relieve discomfort, it is no more likely to produce a cure for these patients than is conventional medicine. Patients end up on an endless merry-go-round of chiropractic adjustments, or miracle supplements, or special diets.

The only cure for somaticized symptoms is to deal with the source directly. We must accept our psychological pain and face it. When we are able to experience our anger, or our depression, or anxiety, or loss and heal them at the level of our feelings, then the need for our physical symptoms will disappear.

This can be profoundly difficult to do. It can be troubling to even consider the possibility that our emotions may be influencing our health. If you have one of the conditions above, or if you suffer from vague, shifting symptoms that seem to have no medical cause, I would urge you to explore the possibility that you may be somaticizing a psychological conflict. One resource that can be very helpful is <u>The Mind-Body Prescription</u>, by John Sarno, M.D. Counseling, especially Christian counseling, can also be deeply healing.

As we explore the world of alternative medicine, we should always remember that as Christians we have something to give as well as receive. Conventional medicine is a magnificent product of the scientific method, but it offers physical healing with the mind and spirit stripped away. Alternative medicine addresses the hunger for a worldview unconstrained by materialism, and the hunger for deep healing of the whole self, but frequently it also asks us to sacrifice our rationality.

Only the Gospel can reconcile these tensions. In response to conventional medicine, Christianity announces that the world is fundamentally knowable but that there is far more to reality than matter. In response to alternative medicine, the Faith confirms that human beings are dynamic wholes, matter and spirit in union, but it also reminds us that there is One God and One Truth.

Truth is a need. We need truth as much as we need air or water or food. People need to know where they stand in regard to the frequently baffling world in which they find themselves. They also need to know that they can be saved, not just from illness, but from all the evils which surround them, and most especially the evil in their own hearts. Only the Gospel can meet these needs. When we seek healing from either a conventional physician or an alternative practitioner, we must remember that they need healing too, and that we know the proper medicine. Only Christ can heal our deepest wounds.

THE END

WORKS CITED

Agarwal, J.K., and P.K. Nigam. "Achrochordon: a Cutaneous Sign of Carbohydrate Intolerance." <u>Australasian Journal of Dermatology</u> 28.3 (1987): 132-3.

Alpha Tocopherol, Beta Carotene Cancer Prevention Study Group. "The Effect of Vitamin E and Beta Carotene on the Incidence of Lung Cancer and Other Cancers in Male Smokers." <u>New England Journal of Medicine</u> 330 (1994): 1029-35.

Assendelft, Willem J.J., M.D., et al. "The Relationship Between Methodological Quality and Conclusions in Reviews of Spinal Manipulation." <u>JAMA</u> 274 (1995): 1942-7.

Astin, John A. "Why Patients Use Alternative Medicine: Results of a National Study." <u>JAMA</u> 279 (1998): 1548-53.

Bennett, William, M.D., and Joel Gurin. <u>The Dieter's Dilemma: Eating Less and Weighing More</u>. New York: Basic Books, 1982.

Benson, Herbert. "Should You Consult Dr. God?" <u>Prevention</u> December 1996: 60-67.

Bone, M.E., et al. "Ginger Root—A New Antiemetic. The Effect of Ginger Root on Postoperative Nausea and Vomiting After Major Gynaecological Surgery." <u>Anaesthesia</u> 45 (1990): 669-71.

Bonhoeffer, Dietrich. <u>Letters and Papers from Prison</u>. Eberhard Bethage, ed. Reginald H. Fuller, trans. New York: The Macmillan Company, 1953.

Bratman, Steven, and David Kroll, eds. Natural Health Bible. Rocklin, CA: Prima, 1999.

Carey, T.S., et al. "The Outcomes and Costs of Care for Acute Low Back Pain Among Patients Seen by Primary Care Practitioners, Chiropractors, and Orthopedic Surgeons. The North Carolina Back Pain Project." New England Journal of Medicine 333 (1995): 913-7.

Cassileth, B.R., et al. "Survival and Quality of Life Among Patients Receiving Unproven as Compared With Conventional Cancer Therapy." New England Journal of Medicine 324 (1991): 1180-5.

Catechism of the Catholic Church. Ligouri, MO: Ligouri Publications, 1994.

Chandra, R.K. "Effect of Vitamin and Trace-element Supplementation on Immune Responses and Infection in Elderly Subjects." Lancet 340.8828 (1992): 1124-7.

Chao, D.M., et al. "Naloxone Reverses Inhibitory Effect of Electroacupuncture on Sympathetic Cardiovascular Reflex Responses." American Journal of Physiology 276.6 Pt 2 (1999): H2127-34.

Christensen, Larry. Diet-Behavior Relationships: Focus on Depression. Washington, D.C.: American Psychological Association, 1996.

"Coenzyme Q10: The Next Aspirin?" Harvard Heart Letter February 1996: 5-7.

Corr, L.A., and M.F. Oliver. "The Low Fat/Low Cholesterol Diet is Ineffective." European Heart Journal 18 (1997): 18-22.

Coulter, Harris L., Ph.D. Homoeopathic Science and Modern Medicine. Berkeley: North Atlantic Books, 1981.

Dabbs, V., and W.J. Lauretti. "A Risk Assessment of Cervical Manipulation vs. NSAIDs for the Treatment of Neck Pain." <u>Journal of Manipulative and Physiological Therapeutics</u> 18 (1995): 530-6.

Efendy, J.L., et al. "The Effect of the Aged Garlic Extract, 'Kyolic', on the Development of Experimental Atherosclerosis." <u>Atherosclerosis</u> 132 (1997): 37-42.

Eisenberg, David, M.D., with Thomas Lee Wright. <u>Encounters With Qi: Exploring Chinese Medicine</u>. New York: W.W. Norton and Company, 1995.

Enstrom, J.E., L.E. Kanim, and M.A. Klein. "Vitamin C Intake and Mortality Among a Sample of the United States Population." <u>Epidemiology</u> 3.3 (1992): 194-202.

Flora, K., et al. "Milk Thistle (Silybum Marianum) for the Therapy of Liver Disease." <u>American Journal of Gastroenterology</u> 93.2 (1998): 139-43.

Friedman, Tracey, et al. "Use of Alternative Therapies for Children With Cancer." <u>Pediatrics</u> 100.6 (1997): e1. http://www.pediatrics.org

Fugh-Berman, Adriane, M.D. <u>Alternative Medicine: What Works</u>. Tucson: Odonian Press, 1996.

Gerber, Suzanne. "What's Love Got to Do With It?" <u>Vegetarian Times</u> n. 247 (1998): 62-66.

Grossinger, Richard. <u>Homeopathy: An Introduction for Skeptics and Beginners</u>. Berkeley: North Atlantic Books, 1993.

Hemila, H. "Does Vitamin C Alleviate the Symptoms of the Common Cold?—A Review of Current Evidence." <u>Scandinavian Journal of Infectious Diseases</u> 26.1 (1994): 1-6.

Hennekins, Charles H., et al. "Lack of Effect of Long-term Supplementation With Beta Carotene on the Incidence of Malignant Neoplasms and Cardiovascular Disease." New England Journal of Medicine 334 (1996): 1145-9.

Homocysteine Lowering Trialists' Collaboration. "Lowering Blood Homocysteine With Folic Acid Based Supplements: Meta-analysis of Randomized Trials." BMJ 316 (1998): 894-8.

Houston, D.K., et al. "Individual Foods and Food Group Patterns of the Oldest Old." Journal of Nutrition for the Elderly 13.4 (1994): 5-23.

Hunick, M.G., et al. "The Recent Decline in Mortality from Coronary Heart Disease, 1980-1990. The Effect of Secular Trends in Risk Factors and Treatment." JAMA 277 (1997): 535-42.

Hurwitz, E.L., et al. "Manipulation and Mobilization of the Cervical Spine. A Systematic Review of the Literature." Spine 21 (1996): 1746-60.

Jacobs, Jennifer, et al. "Treatment of Acute Childhood Diarrhea With Homeopathic Medicine: A Randomized Clinical Trial in Nicaragua." Pediatrics 93 (1994): 719-25.

Kahn, H.A., and T.R. Dawber. "The Development of Coronary Heart Disease in Relation to Sequential Biennial Measures of Cholesterol in the Framingham Study." Journal of Chronic Diseases 19.5 (1966): 611-20.

Keys, Ancel, et al. "Epidemiological Studies Related to Coronary Heart Disease: Characteristics of Men Aged 40-59 in Seven Countries." Acta Medica Scandinavica Supplement 460 (1966): 1-392.

Kingston, Maxine Hong. China Men. New York: Ballantine, 1980.

Kleijnen, Jos, Paul Knipschild, and Gerben ter Riet. "Clinical Trials of Homeopathy." BMJ 302 (1991): 316-23.

Knaster, Mirka. "Matthew Fox, Radical Priest." EastWest Natural Health January/February 1992: 21-24.

Koscielny, J., et al. "The Antiatherosclerotic Effect of Allium Sativum." Atherosclerosis 144 (1999): 237-49.

Le Bars, P.L., et al. "A Placebo-controlled, Double-blind, Randomized Trial of an Extract of Ginkgo Biloba for Dementia. North American Egb Study Group." JAMA 278 (1997): 1327-32.

Lindahl, O., and L. Lindwall. "Double Blind Study of a Valerian Preparation." Pharmacology, Biochemistry, and Behavior 32 (1989): 1065-6.

Linde, K., et al. "Are the Clinical Effects of Homeopathy Placebo Effects? A Meta-analysis of Placebo-controlled Trials." Lancet 350.9081 (1997): 834-43.

Losonczy, Katalin G., Tamara B. Harris, and Richard J. Havlik. "Vitamin E and Vitamin C Supplement Use and Risk of All-cause and Coronary Heart Disease Mortality in Older Persons: the Established Populations for Epidemiologic Studies of the Elderly." American Journal of Clinical Nutrition 64.2 (1996): 190-6.

Manton, K.G., L. Corder, and E. Stallard. "Chronic Disability Trends in Elderly United States Populations: 1982-1994." National Academy of Sciences of the United States of America. Proceedings 94 (1997): 2593-8.

Mauskop, A., and B.M. Altura. "Role of Magnesium in the Pathogenesis and Treatment of Migraines." Clinical Neuroscience 5 (1998): 24-7.

Maxwell, Joe. "Nursing's New Age?" <u>Christianity Today</u> 5 February 1996: 96-99.

McAlindon, Timothy E., et al. "Glucosamine and Chondroitin for Treatment of Osteoarthritis: A Systematic Quality Assessment and Meta-analysis." <u>JAMA</u> 283 (2000): 1469-75.

Moore, J. Stuart. <u>Chiropractic in America: The History of a Medical Alternative</u>. Baltimore: The Johns Hopkins UP, 1993.

Moore, Thomas J. <u>Lifespan: Who Lives Longer and Why</u>. New York: Simon and Schuster, 1993.

Omen, Gilbert S., et al. "Effects of a Combination of Beta Carotene and Vitamin A on Lung Cancer and Cardiovascular Disease." <u>New England Journal of Medicine</u> 334 (1996): 1150-55.

Ornish, Dean, et al. "Intensive Lifestyle Changes for Reversal of Coronary Heart Disease." <u>JAMA</u> 280 (1998): 2001-7.

Plosker, G.L., and R.N. Brogden. "Serenoa Repens (Permixon). A Review of Its Pharmacology and Therapeutic Efficacy in Benign Prostatic Hyperplasia." <u>Drugs and Aging</u> 9.5 (1996): 379-95.

Reaven, Gerald, and A. Laws. "Insulin Resistance, Compensatory Hyperinsulinaemia, and Coronary Heart Disease." <u>Diabetologia</u> 37 (1994): 948-52.

Reddy, Marlita A., ed. <u>Statistical Abstract of the World</u>. Detroit: Gale, 1994.

Reilly, David, et al. "Is Evidence for Homoeopathy Reproducible?" <u>Lancet</u> 344.8937 (1994): 1601-6.

Reston, James. "Now, About My Operation in Peking." <u>New York Times</u> 26 July 1971, late city edition: 1,6.

Rothstein, William G. "The Botanical Movements and Orthodox Medicine" in Other Healers: Unorthodox Medicine in America. Norman Gevitz, ed. Baltimore: Johns Hopkins UP, 1988. 29-51.

Sarno, John. The MindBody Prescription. New York: Warner Books, 1999.

Seddon, J.M., et al. "The Use of Vitamin Supplements and the Risk of Cataract Among US Male Physicians." American Journal of Public Health 84 (1994): 788-92.

Sneed, Dr. David and Dr. Sharon Sneed. The Hidden Agenda: A Critical View of Alternative Medical Therapies. Nashville: Thomas Nelson, 1991.

Soja, A.M., and S.A. Mortensen. "Treatment of Congestive Heart Failure With Coenzyme Q10 Illuminated by Meta-analysis of Clinical Trials." Molecular Aspects of Medicine 18.Supplement (1997): S159-68.

Stampfer, M.J., et al. "Vitamin E Consumption and the Risk of Coronary Disease in Women." New England Journal of Medicine 328 (1993): 1444-9.

Stephens, N.G., et al. "Randomized Controlled Trial of Vitamin E in Patients With Coronary Disease: Cambridge Heart Antioxidant Study (CHAOS)." Lancet 347.9004 (1996): 781-6.

Virju, A. "A Study of Patients Attending Without Appointments in an Urban General Practice." BMJ 301.6742 (1990): 22-6.

Wang, D.C. "Influence of Astragalus Membranaceus Polysaccharide FB on Immunologic Function of Human Periphery Blood Lymphocyte (English abstract)." Chung Hua Chung Liu Tsa Chih 11.3 (1989): 180-3.

Wang, S.Y., et al. "The Anti-tumor Effect of Ganoderma Lucidum is Mediated by Cytokines Released from Activated Macrophages and T Lymphocytes." International Journal of Cancer 70.6 (1997): 699-705.

Weil, Andrew, M.D. Health and Healing. Boston: Houghton Mifflin, 1988.

Weiss, Rudolf Fritz, M.D. Herbal Medicine. A.R. Meuss, trans. Beaconsfield, England: Beaconsfield Publishers Ltd., 1994.

Williams, Dr. Roger J. Nutrition Against Disease. New York: Bantam, 1978.

Wolfe, M.M. "NSAIDs and the Gastrointestinal Mucosa." Hospital Practice 31.12 (1996): 37-44, 47-8.

Wurtman, Judith, et al. "The Effect of a Carbohydrate-rich Beverage on Mood, Appetite, and Cognitive Function in Women With Premenstrual Syndrome." Obstetrics and Gynecology 86.4 Pt 1 (1995): 520-8.

Wyatt, Katrina M., et al. "Efficacy of Vitamin B-6 in the Treatment of Premenstrual Syndrome: Systematic Review." BMJ 318 (1999): 1375-81.

0-595-26568-5